Clinical Practice Guideline

Number 15

Treatment of Pressure Ulcers

Treatment of Pressure Ulcers Guideline Panel

Nancy Bergstrom, PhD, RN, FAAN (Chair)
Richard M. Allman, MD
Oscar M. Alvarez, PhD
M. Alisan Bennett, EdD, RN
Carolyn E. Carlson, PhD, RN
Rita A. Frantz, PhD, RN, FAAN
Susan L. Garber, MA, OTR, FAOTA
Bettie S. Jackson, EdD, MBA, FAAN
Mitchell V. Kaminski, Jr., MD, SC, FACS, FICS, FACN
Mildred G. Kemp, PhD, RN, CETN, FAAN
Thomas A. Krouskop, PhD
Victor L. Lewis, Jr., MD, FACS
JoAnn Maklebust, MSN, RN, CS
David J. Margolis, MD, FACP
Elena M. Marvel, MSN, MA, RN
Steven I. Reger, PhD, CP
George T. Rodeheaver, PhD
Richard Salcido, MD, FAAPMR
George C. Xakellis, MD
Gary M. Yarkony, MD, FAAPMR

U.S. Department of Health and Human Services
Public Health Service
Agency for Health Care Policy and Research
Rockville, Maryland

AHCPR Publication No. 95-0652
December 1994

Guideline Development and Use

Guidelines are systematically developed statements to assist practitioner and patient decisions about appropriate health care for specific clinical conditions. This guideline was developed by a private-sector panel convened by the Agency for Health Care Policy and Research (AHCPR). The panel employed an explicit, science-based methodology and expert clinical judgment to develop specific statements on patient assessment and management for the clinical condition selected.

Extensive literature searches were conducted and critical reviews and syntheses were used to evaluate empirical evidence and significant outcomes. Peer review and field review were undertaken to evaluate the validity, reliability, and utility of the guideline in clinical practice. The panel's recommendations are primarily based on the published scientific literature. When the scientific literature was incomplete or inconsistent in a particular area, the recommendations reflect the professional judgment of panel members and consultants.

The guideline reflects the state of knowledge, current at the time of publication, on effective and appropriate care. Given the inevitable changes in the state of scientific information and technology, periodic review, updating, and revision will be done.

We believe that the AHCPR-assisted clinical practice guidelines will make positive contributions to the quality of care in the United States. We encourage practitioners and patients to use the information provided in this *Clinical Practice Guideline.* The recommendations may not be appropriate for use in all circumstances. Decisions to adopt any particular recommendation must be made by the practitioner in light of available resources and circumstances presented by individual patients.

Clifton R. Gaus, ScD
Administrator
Agency for Health Care Policy and Research

Publication of this guideline does not necessarily represent endorsement by the U.S. Department of Health and Human Services.

Foreword

The incidence of pressure ulcers is sufficiently high, especially among certain high-risk groups, to warrant concern among health care providers. These groups include elderly patients admitted to the hospital for femoral fracture (66-percent incidence) and critical care patients (33-percent incidence). In addition, the prevalence of pressure ulcers in skilled care facilities and nursing homes is reported to be as high as 23 percent. An extensive study of acute care facilities reported a prevalence of 9.2 percent, and in one study of quadriplegic patients the prevalence was 60 percent.

Because prevention of this debilitating condition is believed to be less costly than its treatment, the panel initially produced a guideline entitled, *Pressure Ulcers in Adults: Prediction and Prevention. Clinical Practice Guideline, No. 3*. Although it is certainly desirable to prevent pressure ulcers, individuals still enter the health care system with ulcers or develop ulcers during periods of increased vulnerability as their physical condition deteriorates. This guideline addresses the treatment of pressure ulcers. It is intended for clinicians who examine and treat persons with pressure ulcers, and the treatment recommendations focus on (1) assessment of the patient and pressure ulcer, (2) tissue load management, (3) ulcer care, (4) management of bacterial colonization and infection, (5) operative repair, and (6) education and quality improvement.

AHCPR appointed an external panel of multidisciplinary experts in this field to develop the guideline. To provide a scientific basis for this guideline, the panel conducted comprehensive literature searches, reviewed more than 45,000 abstracts, evaluated approximately 1,700 papers, and cited 333 references to support this guideline.

The panel solicited input from a broad array of organizations and individuals. Testimony was provided by interested parties at a public forum on April 9, 1992, in Washington, DC. A draft of the guideline was distributed to and analyzed by participants at a conference sponsored by the National Pressure Ulcer Advisory Panel and the Wound Ostomy and Continence Nurses Society in March 1993. The Treatment of Pressure Ulcers Guideline Panel also invited peer review by individual experts, professional organizations, consumers, and Government regulatory agencies. Health care agencies conducted pilot reviews to evaluate the clinical applicability of the guideline. In all, more than 400 reviewers have critiqued various drafts of this guideline.

This first edition of *Treatment of Pressure Ulcers* will be periodically revised and updated as needed so that future editions reflect new research findings and experience with emerging technologies and innovative approaches. To this end, the panel welcomes comments and suggestions regarding the current guideline. Please send written comments to Director, Office of the Forum for Quality and Effectiveness in Health Care, AHCPR, 6000 Executive Boulevard, Suite 310, Rockville, MD 20852.

Treatment of Pressure Ulcers Guideline Panel

Abstract

This *Clinical Practice Guideline* offers a comprehensive program for treating adults with pressure ulcers. The recommendations are intended for clinicians who examine and treat individuals in all health care settings.

The guideline was developed by a panel of experts and is based on the best available scientific evidence and clinical expertise. The recommended treatment program focuses on (1) assessment of the patient and pressure ulcer, (2) tissue load management, (3) ulcer care, (4) management of bacterial colonization and infection, (5) operative repair in selected patients with Stage III and IV pressure ulcers, and (6) education and quality improvement.

Accurate, ongoing assessment of the ulcer is essential. Of equal importance are the assessment and management of the individual's overall health, including physical, psychosocial, and nutritional status. Pain should be assessed and managed. Management of tissue loads (i.e., pressure, friction, and shear), through vigilant use of positioning techniques and appropriately selected support surfaces, is critical.

Ulcer care includes (1) debridement of necrotic tissue and debris, (2) wound cleansing using saline and avoiding antiseptics, and (3) application of dressings that maintain a clean, moist environment while keeping the surrounding skin dry. Education and quality improvement are integral to an effective pressure ulcer treatment program.

Bergstrom N, Bennett MA, Carlson CE, et al. *Treatment of Pressure Ulcers.* Clinical Practice Guideline, No. 15. Rockville, MD: U.S. Department of Health and Human Services. Public Health Service, Agency for Health Care Policy and Research. AHCPR Publication No. 95–0652. December 1994.

Panel Members

Nancy Bergstrom, PhD, RN, FAAN
Panel Chair, 1991–94
Professor and Interim Associate Dean
Graduate Nursing Programs
University of Nebraska Medical Center
Omaha, Nebraska
Specialty: Pressure Ulcer Research

Richard M. Allman, MD
Panelist, 1991–92
Consultant, 1992–94
Associate Professor of Medicine
Director of the Center for Aging and the Division of Gerontology and Geriatrics
University of Alabama at Birmingham
Chief of Geriatrics Section
Birmingham Department of Veterans Affairs Medical Center
Birmingham, Alabama
Specialty: Geriatric Medicine

Oscar M. Alvarez, PhD
1991–92
Director
University Wound Healing Clinic
New Brunswick, New Jersey
Specialty: Wound Healing

M. Alisan Bennett, EdD, RN
1993–94
Supervisor and Special Projects Coordinator
Nursing Education and Research
Woodhull Medical and Mental Health Center of the New York City Health and Hospitals Corporation
Brooklyn, New York
Specialty: Preservation of Darkly Pigmented Intact Skin

Carolyn E. Carlson, PhD, RN
1991–94
Professor of Nursing
Cedarville College
Cedarville, Ohio
Associate Director of Nursing and Allied Health for Research and Evaluation, Division of Nursing and Allied Health, and Department of Research
Rehabilitation Institute of Chicago
Chicago, Illinois
Specialty: Rehabilitation and Psychiatric Nursing

Rita A. Frantz, PhD, RN, FAAN
1991–94
Associate Professor
College of Nursing
University of Iowa
Clinical Associate in Nursing
Iowa Veterans Home
Iowa City, Iowa
Specialty: Wound Care

Susan L. Garber, MA, OTR, FAOTA
1991–94
Assistant Director for Research and Education
Department of Occupational Therapy
The Institute for Rehabilitation and Research
Assistant Professor
Department of Physical Medicine and Rehabilitation
Baylor College of Medicine
Houston, Texas
Specialty: Occupational Therapy

Bettie S. Jackson, EdD, MBA, FAAN
1991–94
Director of Professional Services
Department of Nursing
Moses Division, Montefiore Medical Center
Bronx, New York
Associate Research Scientist
School of Nursing
Columbia University
New York, New York
Specialty: Administration and Enterostomal Therapy

Mitchell V. Kaminski, Jr., MD, SC, FACS, FICS, FACN
1991–94
Staff Surgeon
Thorek Hospital and Medical Center
Clinical Professor of Surgery
Chicago Medical School
University of Health Sciences
Chicago, Illinois
Specialty: Surgery and Nutritional Support

Mildred G. Kemp, PhD, RN, CETN, FAAN
1991–94
Associate Professor
College of Nursing
Rush University
Practitioner/Teacher
Department of Operating Room and Surgical Nursing
Rush-Presbyterian-St. Luke's Medical Center
Chicago, Illinois
Specialty: Enterostomal Therapy

Thomas A. Krouskop, PhD
1991–92
Professor
Department of Physical Medicine and Rehabilitation
Baylor College of Medicine
Director of Rehabilitation Engineering
The Institute for Rehabilitation and Research
Houston, Texas
Specialty: Bioengineering

Victor L. Lewis, Jr., MD, FACS
1991–94
Associate Professor of Clinical Surgery
Northwestern University Medical School
Chicago, Illinois
Specialty: Plastic Surgery

JoAnn Maklebust, MSN, RN, CS
1991–94
Clinical Nurse Specialist, Wound Care
Case Manager, General and Reconstructive Surgery
Harper Hospital
Detroit Medical Center
Detroit, Michigan
Specialty: Wound Care

David J. Margolis, MD, FACP
1992–94
Director
Cutaneous Ulcer Center
University of Pennsylvania Medical Center
Assistant Professor
Department of Dermatology
School of Medicine
University of Pennsylvania
Philadelphia, Pennsylvania
Specialty: Dermatology

Elena M. Marvel, MSN, MA, RN
1991–94
State Coordinator
Health Advocacy Services Program in New Jersey
American Association of Retired Persons
Short Hills, New Jersey
Specialty: Consumer Advocacy

Steven I. Reger, PhD, CP
1992–94
Director of Rehabilitation Engineering
Department of Physical Medicine and Rehabilitation
Department of Plastic Surgery
Department of Biomedical Engineering
The Cleveland Clinic Foundation
Cleveland, Ohio
Specialty: Biomedical Engineering

George T. Rodeheaver, PhD
Panelist, 1991–92
Consultant, 1992–94
Professor and Director
Plastic Surgery Research
Health Sciences Center
University of Virginia
Charlottesville, Virginia
Specialty: Wound Management Research

Richard Salcido, MD, FAAPMR
1993–94
Interim Chairman
Department of Physical Medicine and Rehabilitation
Associate
Department of BioMedical Engineering
Associate
Sanders-Brown Center on Aging
University of Kentucky
Cardinal Hill Hospital
Lexington, Kentucky
Specialty: Physical Medicine and Rehabilitation

George C. Xakellis, MD
1991–94
Director of Research and Medical Development
John Deere Health Care Corporation
Moline, Illinois
Specialty: Family Medicine

Gary M. Yarkony, MD, FAAPMR
1992–94
Vice President for Clinical Development
Schwab Rehabilitation Hospital and Care Network
Associate Professor of Clinical Physical Medicine and Rehabilitation
Northwestern University Medical School
Chicago, Illinois
Specialty: Physical Medicine and Rehabilitation

Acknowledgments

Many organizations and individuals made significant contributions during the development of this guideline. Although they are too numerous to mention here, the Contributors section, which appears later in this publication, lists individual consultants, peer reviewers, and support staff. This guideline would not have been possible without their collaborative efforts.

All persons, organizations, and agencies with an interest in the pressure ulcer treatment guideline were invited to participate at a public meeting held in Washington, DC, on April 9, 1992, and the panel gratefully acknowledges the valuable input received during that session.

The National Pressure Ulcer Advisory Panel (NPUAP) and the Wound, Ostomy, and Continence Nurses Society (WOCN) are to be commended for their ongoing efforts to improve the prevention and treatment of pressure ulcers. George T. Rodeheaver, PhD, president of the NPUAP, deserves special recognition for his efforts in mobilizing the NPUAP's resources to provide a forum for peer review of the pressure ulcer treatment guideline. Input from participants attending the jointly sponsored NPUAP and WOCN meeting on March 5–6, 1993, was extremely helpful.

Product manufacturers also contributed to the guideline development process. Many companies responded to requests for published and unpublished information regarding the results of product research. The panel appreciates their contributions.

The panel gratefully acknowledges the supportive efforts of Margaret Coopey, MGA, RN, project officer from the Office of the Forum for Quality and Effectiveness in Health Care, AHCPR, and of William N. LeVee (managing editor) and Karen Carp (product manager) from the Center for Research Dissemination and Liaison, AHCPR.

The panel also extends its gratitude and appreciation to the support staff members for their tireless efforts: Janet Cuddigan, PhC, RN, panel manager, research analyst, and scientific writer; Brenda Bergman-Evans, PhD, RNC, research analyst and scientific writer; Joan Ronnenberg, MSN, RN, research analyst; Elizabeth Gavin, panel secretary; Joyce Black, MSN, RN, scientific writer; and Diane Q. Forti, BA, scientific editor.

Heartfelt gratitude is extended to the families of panel members for their patience, support, and understanding. This guideline is dedicated to the patients we are privileged to serve.

Contents

Tables

Figures

Executive Summary

Background

Pressure ulcers can be a common and costly problem in acute care, nursing home, and home care populations. For example, the incidence (new cases appearing within a specified period of time) of pressure ulcers in acute care facilities has ranged from 2.7 to 29.5 percent. Prevalence (a cross-sectional count of the number of cases at a specified point in time) in this setting has varied between 3.5 and 29.5 percent. Several populations may be at even higher risk, including quadriplegic patients (60-percent prevalence), elderly patients admitted for femoral fracture (66-percent incidence), and critical care patients (33-percent incidence and 41-percent prevalence). Studies conducted in skilled care facilities and nursing homes have indicated prevalence rates ranging between 2.4 and 23 percent. In a recent 1-year study of 326 home health care patients, the incidence of pressure ulcers was 4.3 percent and the prevalence was 12.9 percent.

In economic terms, the reported cost of pressure ulcer treatment can vary greatly. Miller and Delozier estimated that the total national cost of pressure ulcer treatment exceeds $1.335 billion. Implementation of the recommendations of this guideline is estimated to reduce the cost of pressure ulcer treatment by 3 percent or $40 million.

The panel anticipates that its earlier guideline, *Pressure Ulcers in Adults: Prediction and Prevention. Clinical Practice Guideline, No. 3,* will stimulate the development of effective prevention programs, thereby reducing the incidence of pressure ulcers. Unfortunately, not all pressure ulcers will be prevented and those that do develop may become chronic. Therefore, this pressure ulcer treatment guideline offers recommendations for the effective treatment of pressure ulcers in adults. At the clinician's discretion, the recommendations in this guideline may also be applied to children, but not to neonates.

Definitions

A pressure ulcer is any lesion caused by unrelieved pressure resulting in damage of underlying tissue. Pressure ulcers usually occur over bony prominences and are graded or staged to classify the degree of tissue damage observed. Stage I pressure ulcers are defined as nonblanchable erythema of intact skin. (Although Stage I pressure ulcers are not the focus of this treatment guideline, their appearance should prompt greater vigilance in implementing preventive strategies.) Stage II is defined as partial thickness skin loss involving epidermis, dermis, or both. Stage III is characterized by full thickness skin loss involving damage or necrosis of subcutaneous tissue that may extend down to, but not through, underlying fascia. Stage IV pressure ulcers show full thickness skin loss with extensive destruction, tissue necrosis, or damage to muscle, bone, or supporting structures.

When assessing a pressure ulcer, one should consider the following limitations in the preceding definitions: (1) It may be difficult to detect Stage I pressure ulcers in darkly pigmented skin; (2) when eschar is present, accurate staging is not possible until the eschar has been removed; and (3) pressure ulcers under casts, orthopedic devices, and support stockings are difficult to assess and require extra diligence.

Guideline Development

To develop this guideline, AHCPR convened a multidisciplinary private-sector panel of physicians, nurses, an occupational therapist, a biomedical engineer, and a consumer representative. In developing the scientific base to support guideline recommendations, the panel conducted an extensive review of the literature on pressure ulcers in adults, heard public testimony at an open forum, examined information obtained from consultants, and submitted several guideline drafts for peer and pilot review.

The panel considered a broad range of interventions including accurate, ongoing assessment of the patient and the ulcer; management of pressure, friction, and shear through the use of specific positioning techniques and support surfaces; care of the ulcer, including debridement, cleansing, dressings, and selected adjunctive therapies; measures to control bacterial colonization and treat infection; operative repair of the ulcers; patient and caregiver education; and quality improvement programs. The scientific evidence, benefits, and harms associated with each intervention were examined using established criteria to rate the strength of evidence. The intent of the panel was to recommend those interventions that were supported by at least one controlled trial. In reality, many well-established clinical practices have never been investigated experimentally. The strength-of-evidence rating printed after the panel recommendations cues the reader to the level of support associated with each recommendation. The known harms of each intervention were carefully identified, and interventions were recommended only if the benefits clearly outweighed potential harms.

Target Audience

The *Clinical Practice Guideline* recommendations are intended for clinicians who examine and treat persons who have pressure ulcers. Therefore, the guideline will be of interest to family physicians, internists, geriatricians, physiatrists, nurses and nurse practitioners, enterostomal therapists, infection control officers, physical and occupational therapists, psychological support staff, and dietitians in acute care, long-term care, rehabilitative, geriatric, and home settings. In addition, the recommendations may be useful to health care administrators, policy analysts, regulatory agencies, and third-party payers. Because patients and families are integral to the management team in all settings and during all phases of treatment, they should be apprised of the benefits and harms of available treatment options. Treatments should be consistent with patient goals, values, and personal preferences. Recommendations are applicable to patients seeking palliative as well as restorative care.

Guideline Recommendations

This pressure ulcer treatment guideline provides specific recommendations in six areas described subsequently in detail.

- Assessment.
- Managing tissue loads.
- Ulcer care.
- Managing bacterial colonization and infection.
- Operative repair.
- Education and quality improvement.

Assessment

The assessment of an individual with a pressure ulcer is the basis for planning treatment, evaluating treatment effects, and communicating with other caregivers. Initially, the clinician should determine the location, stage, and size of the pressure ulcer and whether sinus tracts, undermining, tunneling, exudate, necrotic tissue, granulation tissue, and epithelialization are present. Pressure ulcers should be assessed at least once a week, but deterioration either in the patient's overall condition or in the pressure ulcer itself mandates more immediate reassessment as well as a reevaluation of the treatment plan. Clinicians can reasonably expect a clean pressure ulcer with adequate innervation and blood supply to show evidence of healing within 2 to 4 weeks. Failure to do so should prompt a reevaluation of the plan of care, an evaluation of adherence to the plan, and a possible modification of the plan.

In developing a pressure ulcer treatment plan, the clinician should assess not only the pressure ulcer but also the entire person. Such an assessment should include (1) a complete history and physical examination, (2) the identification of complications and comorbid conditions, (3) a nutritional assessment, (4) an assessment of pain, (5) a psychosocial assessment, and (6) an evaluation of the individual's risks for additional pressure ulcers.

The history and physical examination will help the clinician understand the patient's overall physical and psychosocial health. Special attention should be directed to identification and management of illnesses that might impede healing, such as peripheral vascular disease, diabetes mellitus, immune deficiencies, collagen vascular diseases, malignancies, psychosis, and depression. Complications known to be associated with pressure ulcers should be identified and treated early. Possible complications include amyloidosis, endocarditis, heterotopic bone formation, maggot infestation, meningitis, perineal–urethral fistula, pseudoaneurysm, septic arthritis, sinus tract or abscess, squamous cell carcinoma in the ulcer, systemic effects of topical treatments (e.g., iodine toxicity), osteomyelitis, bacteremia, sepsis, and advancing cellulitis.

Nutritional assessment and management are essential to any successful pressure ulcer treatment program. A patient with pressure ulcers should undergo a nutritional assessment, with nutritional status reassessed periodically according to the patient's condition. The panel recommends the 1991 *Nutrition Screening Manual* as a guide for nutritional assessment. The stage of an existing pressure ulcer has been found to correlate with the severity of nutritional deficits, especially low dietary protein intake and hypoalbuminemia. In addition, studies have demonstrated an association between malnutrition and the development of new pressure ulcers. Risk factors for malnutrition include the inability to take food by mouth or a history of an involuntary change in weight. For individuals at risk for malnutrition, an abbreviated nutritional assessment should be conducted at least every 3 months. Clinicians should encourage dietary intake and supplementation in pressure ulcer patients who are malnourished. If dietary intake remains inadequate, nutritional support (such as tube feeding) should be provided if this is consistent with the goals of care. Approximately 30 to 35 calories/kg/day and 1.25 to 1.50 grams of protein/kg/day are recommended to place the patient in positive nitrogen balance. If deficiencies are demonstrated or suspected, vitamin and mineral supplements should be given. Caregivers should ensure an adequate dietary intake to the extent compatible with the patient's wishes.

Although research related to the assessment of pressure ulcer pain is surprisingly scarce, the panel recommends that clinicians routinely assess for pain, recognizing that pain may be intensified during dressing changes and debridement. Pain should be managed by eliminating or controlling its source and providing analgesia. Further research needs to be conducted to identify the most effective methods of assessing and managing pain associated with pressure ulcers.

A psychosocial assessment should be carried out to determine whether the patient comprehends the treatment program and is motivated to adhere to it. This assessment also provides the clinician an excellent opportunity to understand the values, lifestyle, psychosocial needs, and goals of the individual, family, and caregiver and thus collaboratively set treatment goals and arrange interventions that meet the unique needs of the individual. The resources available to individuals being treated at home should also be noted.

Individuals with existing pressure ulcers may be at risk for developing additional ulcers. Risk factors should be identified and modified as part of the treatment regimen (see guideline entitled *Pressure Ulcers in Adults: Prediction and Prevention. Clinical Practice Guideline, No. 3).*

Managing Tissue Loads

The goal of tissue load management is to create an environment that enhances soft tissue viability and promotes healing of the pressure ulcer(s). Specific interventions are designed to decrease the magnitude of pressure, friction, and shear and to provide levels of moisture and temperature that support tissue health and growth. These goals can be met through vigilant use of proper positioning techniques and support surfaces, whether the individual is in bed or sitting in a chair.

While in Bed. Individuals who are in bed should not be positioned on the pressure ulcer(s). If the ulcer is on a circumscribed area such as the heel or the back of the head, positioning devices should be used to raise the ulcer off the support surface. Avoid using donut-type (ring) devices. A written repositioning schedule should be developed and implemented to protect uninvolved areas. The following preventive strategies will benefit patients considered to be at risk for developing additional pressure ulcers:

- Avoid positioning immobile individuals directly on their trochanters.
- Use positioning devices to relieve all pressure from the heels and to prevent direct contact between bony prominences.
- Prevent shear injury by maintaining the head of the bed at the lowest level of elevation and for the shortest period of time that is consistent with medical conditions and other restrictions.

For a more detailed description of these strategies, see the guideline entitled *Pressure Ulcers in Adults: Prediction and Prevention. Clinical Practice Guideline, No. 3.*

A variety of support surfaces can be used to create an environment conducive to healing; however, there is no compelling evidence that one support surface consistently performs better than all others under all circumstances. Support surfaces should be selected with the following performance characteristics in mind: Increased support area, low moisture retention, reduced heat accumulation, shear reduction, pressure reduction, dynamic (versus static) properties, and cost per day. The panel suggests that clinicians consider the following specific recommendations when selecting support surfaces.

- Use pressure-reducing surfaces for individuals at risk for additional ulcers.
- Use a static support surface if the individual can assume a variety of positions without bearing weight on the pressure ulcer and without "bottoming out." To determine if a patient has bottomed out, the

caregiver should place his or her outstretched hand (palm up) under the mattress overlay below the existing pressure ulcer or that part of the body at risk for ulcer formation. If the caregiver can feel that the support material is less than an inch thick at this site, the patient has bottomed out.

- Use a dynamic support surface if the individual is unable to assume a variety of positions without weight bearing on a pressure ulcer, bottoms out on a static support surface, or does not show evidence of healing.
- A low-air-loss or air-fluidized bed may be indicated if a patient has large Stage III or IV pressure ulcers on multiple turning surfaces.
- The drying effect of a low-air-loss or air-fluidized support surface may help prevent additional ulcers when excess moisture on intact skin is identified as a risk factor.

While Sitting. Interface pressure may be particularly high over sitting surfaces. When a pressure ulcer has formed on such a surface, the individual should avoid sitting. If pressure on the ulcer can be totally relieved, the person can sit for a limited time. Proper postural alignment, distribution of weight, balance, stability, and continuous pressure relief are important positioning considerations for the sitting individual. A written plan for the use of positioning devices should be developed and implemented. An individually prescribed seat cushion should be used and donut-type devices should be avoided. Sitting individuals should be repositioned at least every hour and should shift their weight every 15 minutes if possible. If hourly repositioning is not feasible, the individual should be returned to bed.

Ulcer Care

Care of the pressure ulcer itself involves debridement of necrotic tissue, cleansing of the wound at initial examination and at each dressing change, and using a dressing that keeps the ulcer bed continuously moist but the surrounding intact skin dry. Secondarily, adjunctive therapies can be considered.

Debridement. Any necrotic tissue observed during the initial (or subsequent) assessment of the wound should be debrided from the ulcer, if this intervention is consistent with overall patient goals. Because several methods of debridement are available, the clinician should select the method most appropriate to the patient's condition and goals. Regardless of the method selected, the need to assess and control pain should be considered.

Sharp debridement is the most rapid method and may be the most appropriate technique for removing areas of thick, adherent eschar and devitalized tissue in extensive ulcers. When there are signs of advancing cellulitis or sepsis, rapid debridement is imperative, and sharp debridement is the method of choice. Small ulcers may be debrided at the bedside, whereas more extensive ulcers are debrided in the operating room or in special procedures rooms. Sterile instruments should be used, and a clean, dry dressing should be applied for 8 to 24 hours if sharp debridement is associated with bleeding; after 8 to 24 hours, a moist dressing may be resumed. Those who perform sharp debridement should have demonstrated the necessary clinical skills and must meet licensing requirements.

Mechanical debridement includes the use of wet-to-dry dressings at prescribed intervals (usually every 4 to 6 hours), hydrotherapy, wound irrigation, and dextranomers. Wet-to-dry dressings adhere to eschar, removing the eschar when the dry dressing is removed. Because this method tends to be painful and nonselective, adequate analgesia should be provided before dressings are removed, and the clinician should avoid placing a dry dressing over granulating tissue. Hydrotherapy and wound irrigation are useful for softening and mechanically removing eschar and debris. Dextranomers are beads placed in an ulcer bed to absorb exudate, bacteria, and other debris.

Enzymatic debridement is often used in long-term care facilities and in home care. This method of debridement should be considered when the individual cannot tolerate surgery and when the ulcer does not appear to be infected. Infected ulcers should be debrided more rapidly. Enzymatic debridement is accomplished by applying topical debriding agents to devitalized tissue on the wound's surface. Collagenase, a biologic licensed by the Food and Drug Administration (FDA), is an example of such a product. A clean moist dressing should be applied over the ulcer after enzyme application.

Autolytic debridement is accomplished by placing a synthetic dressing over the ulcer and allowing the eschar to self-digest through the action of enzymes normally present in the wound fluid. Although slower than other methods, autolytic debridement may be appropriate for patients who cannot tolerate other methods and are not likely to develop infections. Autolytic debridement is contraindicated in infected ulcers.

Clinicians may elect not to debride heel ulcers that have a dry eschar and no edema, erythema, fluctuance, or drainage. However, these wounds should be assessed daily for complications that might require debridement.

Wound Cleansing. Ulcer wounds should be cleansed initially and at each dressing change. The process of cleansing a wound involves selecting both a wound-cleansing solution and a mechanical means of delivering that solution to the wound. Saline irrigation is a safe and appropriate cleansing method for most pressure ulcers. Antiseptic agents (e.g., povidone iodine, iodophor, sodium hypochlorite solution [Dakin's® solution], hydrogen peroxide, acetic acid) and skin cleansers are toxic to wound tissue and should not be used. Commercial wound cleansers that do not contain harmful chemicals may be used at the clinician's discretion. To avoid traumatizing the wound, the clinician should apply a minimum amount of mechanical force when cleansing with gauze, cloth, or sponges. Irrigation pressures ranging from 4 to 15 pounds per square inch (psi) are safe and effective. For pressure ulcers that contain thick exudate, slough, or necrotic tissue, whirlpool treatment should be considered, but for clean wounds this is not appropriate.

Dressings. Clinicians should select a dressing that will keep the ulcer bed continuously moist while allowing the surrounding intact skin to remain dry. The dressing should control exudate without desiccating the ulcer bed. Caregiver time is a valid consideration when one is selecting a dressing. Although film and hydrocolloid dressings are more expensive than moist saline gauze, the added expense may be offset by savings in caregiver time. Wound dead spaces can be eliminated by loosely filling cavities with dressing materials; overpacking should be avoided. Dressings near the anus are less likely to remain intact and should be carefully monitored.

Adjunctive Therapies. The panel examined the roles of several adjunctive therapies in supporting pressure ulcer healing. These therapies include electrotherapy; hyperbaric oxygen; infrared, ultraviolet, and low-energy laser irradiation; ultrasound; miscellaneous topical agents (including cytokine growth factors); and systemic drugs other than antibiotics. Although many of these therapies hold promise for the future, electrical stimulation is the only adjunctive therapy with sufficient supporting evidence to warrant recommendation at this time. The panel recommends that a course of electrical stimulation be considered for Stage III and IV pressure ulcers that do not respond to conventional therapy.

Managing Bacterial Colonization and Infection

All Stage II, III, and IV pressure ulcers are colonized with bacteria. The panel recommends that colonization be minimized through effective wound cleansing and debridement. If purulence or foul odor develops, more frequent cleansing and possibly debridement are required. Swab cultures should not be used, because they detect only surface colonization and have no diagnostic value. When a culture is required, the Centers for Disease Control and Prevention (CDC) recommend obtaining fluid through needle aspiration or obtaining tissue through ulcer biopsy.

In most cases, adequate cleansing and debridement prevent colonization from progressing to clinical infection. However, if a clean ulcer is not healing or continues to have exudate despite optimal care for 2 to 4 weeks, the clinician should consider a 2-week trial of topical antibiotics that are effective against gram-negative, gram-positive, and anaerobic organisms (e.g., silver sulfadiazine, triple antibiotic).

Healing may be impaired if bacterial levels exceed 10^5 organisms per gram of tissue or if the patient has osteomyelitis. If the ulcer does not respond to topical antibiotic therapy, the clinician should obtain quantitative bacterial cultures, preferably by means of tissue biopsy, and evaluate the underlying bone for osteomyelitis. Topical antiseptics should not be used.

Systemic antibiotics should be given to patients with bacteremia, sepsis, advancing cellulitis, or osteomyelitis but are not required for local pressure ulcer infections.

Pressure ulcers should be protected from exogenous sources of contamination such as feces. In addition, the following infection control measures should be taken to prevent cross-contamination:

- Follow body substance isolation (BSI) precautions or an equivalent isolation system that is appropriate to the setting and the patient's condition.
- Use clean gloves for each patient.
- When treating multiple ulcers on the same patient, attend to the most contaminated ulcer last (e.g., in the perianal region).
- Remove gloves and wash hands between patients.
- Use sterile instruments for debridement.
- Use clean dressings in hospitals, nursing homes, and skilled care facilities to treat pressure ulcers as long as dressing procedures comply with institutional infection control guidelines and appropriate measures are taken to ensure that dressings remain clean when stored.
- Use clean dressings in the home setting if dressings are stored appropriately.
- Follow local regulations to safely dispose of contaminated dressings in the home setting.

Operative Repair

Operative repair should be considered for individuals with clean Stage III or IV pressure ulcers that do not respond to optimal care. Additional research is needed to identify clear criteria for selecting patients most likely to benefit from surgical management. Possible candidates include medically stable patients who are adequately nourished and can tolerate operative blood loss and postoperative immobility. Quality of life, patient preferences, treatment goals, risk of recurrence, and anticipated rehabilitative outcomes should also be considered. Factors that may impair postoperative healing include smoking, spasticity, levels of colonization, incontinence, and urinary tract infection; these should be addressed preoperatively.

Operative procedures include one or more of the following: Direct closure, skin grafting, skin flaps, musculocutaneous flaps, and free flaps. The least traumatic yet most effective method should be selected for ulcer repair. Patients should be counseled on the benefits and harms of the operative techniques appropriate to their circumstances. Prophylactic ischiectomy is not recommended.

Vigilant postoperative followup care is essential to healing. An air-fluidized bed, low-air-loss bed, or Stryker frame should be used for a minimum of 2 weeks postoperatively. Tissue viability at the surgical site should be assessed as clinically indicated. The patient should slowly increase periods of time positioned on the flap to gradually increase tolerance to pressure. As a measure of tolerance, flaps should be monitored to detect pallor or redness that does not resolve after 10 minutes of pressure relief. Patient education and assessment are essential for preventing recurrence.

Education and Quality Improvement

Institutions and health care agencies are responsible for developing and implementing educational programs for patients, families, and caregivers. These programs should translate knowledge about pressure ulcers into effective treatment plans and should cover the entire continuum of care, from prevention through treatments that promote healing and prevent recurrence. Accurate assessment of tissue damage should be emphasized as well as principles of treatment and outcome monitoring. The education program should be an integral part of quality improvement monitoring. In addition, a quality improvement program should be established to facilitate comprehensive, consistent care that can be monitored, evaluated, and changed as conditions warrant.

1 Overview

Introduction

On December 19, 1989, the Omnibus Budget Reconciliation Act (Public Act 101–239) added a new Title IX to the Public Health Service Act establishing the Agency for Health Care Policy and Research (AHCPR). AHCPR's goal is to enhance the quality, appropriateness, and effectiveness of health care services. Section 911 of the Act establishes within AHCPR the Office of the Forum for Quality and Effectiveness in Health Care (the Forum). Section 912 directs the Forum to facilitate the development and periodic review and updating of:

Clinically relevant guidelines that may be used by physicians, educators, and health care practitioners to assist in determining how diseases, disorders, and other health care conditions can most effectively and appropriately be prevented, diagnosed, treated, and managed clinically.

The topic of prediction, prevention, and treatment of pressure ulcers was selected as one of seven topics for initial guideline development based on this mandate, legislative criteria for guideline topics, input from the Nursing Panel for Guideline Development, and the published report of a Consensus Development Conference on pressure ulcers by the National Pressure Ulcer Advisory Panel (NPUAP, 1989). Realizing that prevention of this debilitating condition is less costly than treatment, the panel initially developed *Pressure Ulcers in Adults: Prediction and Prevention. Clinical Practice Guideline, No. 3*. This initial guideline recommended strategies for identifying at-risk individuals, implementing preventive measures, and treating early (Stage I) pressure ulcers. Unfortunately, not all pressure ulcers can be prevented and those that do develop may become chronic. The current guideline provides a comprehensive plan for treating Stage II, III, and IV pressure ulcers. Because individuals with pressure ulcers are at risk for developing additional ulcers, caregivers are encouraged to consider the recommendations offered in the prevention guideline.

The purpose of *Treatment of Pressure Ulcers. Clinical Practice Guideline, No. 15*, is to offer recommendations for the treatment of pressure ulcers. It is intended for clinicians who examine and treat persons with pressure ulcers. Clinicians using this guideline may include family physicians, internists, geriatricians, physiatrists, nurses and nurse practitioners, enterostomal therapists, infection control officers, physical and occupational therapists, psychological support staff, dietitians, and other health care providers working in acute care, long-term care, rehabilitative, geriatric, and home settings. The recommendations may also be useful to health care administrators, policy analysts, regulatory agencies, and third-party payers.

Patients and family caregivers are integral to the management team in all settings and during all phases of treatment. They should be apprised of the benefits and harms of available treatment options. Pressure ulcer treatment should be consistent with patient goals, and patient preferences should be respected. The panel believes that these recommendations are applicable to patients seeking palliative as well as restorative care.

These recommendations are not intended to address any other types of wounds, acute or chronic (e.g., diabetic foot ulcers), or those due to vascular disease (venous stasis or arterial insufficiency), neuropathy, neoplasm, primary skin disease, or thermal or chemical injury. Although these recommendations are based on research involving adults, they may, at the clincian's discretion, be applied to children; however, treatment of neonates may differ from that of children and adults.

The recommended treatment program incorporates (1) assessment of the patient and the pressure ulcer, (2) tissue load management, (3) ulcer care, (4) managing bacterial colonization and infection, (5) operative repair, and (6) education and quality improvement. Although panel members considered a broad range of treatment options, they ultimately recommended only those interventions supported by scientific evidence, expert clinical opinion, or both.

Definitions

A pressure ulcer is any lesion caused by unrelieved pressure resulting in damage of underlying tissue. Pressure ulcers are usually located over bony prominences and are graded or staged to classify the degree of tissue damage observed. Such staging is used as a tool for communication and assessment. The recommendations regarding staging put forth by this panel are consistent with those of the National Pressure Ulcer Advisory Panel Consensus Development Conference (NPUAP, 1989), as derived from previous staging systems proposed by Shea (1975) and the Wound Ostomy and Continence Nurses Society (WOCN) (International Association of Enterostomal Therapy, 1988). Numerical identification of stages does not necessarily imply a progression in ulcer severity. For example, a Stage I ulcer may have very little tissue damage or it may have necrotic underlying tissue, because muscle tissue is more sensitive than skin to pressure-induced ischemia. Pressure ulcers are staged as follows:

Stage I: Nonblanchable erythema of intact skin, the heralding lesion of skin ulceration. In individuals with darker skin, discoloration of the skin, warmth, edema, induration, or hardness may also be indicators.

Stage II: Partial thickness skin loss involving epidermis, dermis, or both. The ulcer is superficial and presents clinically as an abrasion, blister, or shallow crater.

Stage III: Full thickness skin loss involving damage to or necrosis of subcutaneous tissue that may extend down to, but not through, underlying fascia. The ulcer presents clinically as a deep crater with or without undermining of adjacent tissue.

Stage IV: Full thickness skin loss with extensive destruction, tissue necrosis, or damage to muscle, bone, or supporting structures (e.g., tendon, joint capsule). Undermining and sinus tracts also may be associated with Stage IV pressure ulcers.

The following limitations are inherent in these definitions:

1. Because the skin remains intact in Stage I pressure ulcers, these lesions are not ulcers in the usual sense. In addition, Stage I pressure ulcers are not always reliably assessed, especially in patients with darkly pigment ed skin. A reliable system to accurately identify Stage I pressure ulcers in individuals with darkly pigmented skin should be developed. Despite these limitations, identification of a Stage I pressure ulcer is critical for indicating the need for more vigilant assessment and preventive care.

2. When eschar is present, a pressure ulcer cannot be accurately staged until the eschar is removed.

3. It may be difficult to assess pressure ulcers in patients with casts, other orthopedic devices, or support stockings. Routine assessment to check for adequate circulation, movement, and sensation may fail to detect pressure ulcers beneath casts. Health care providers should (1) assess the skin under the edges of casts, (2) be alert to patient complaints of pressure-induced pain, (3) determine whether casts need to be altered or replaced to relieve pressure, and (4) remove support stockings to assess the skin.

Incidence and Prevalence

It has been difficult to determine both the incidence (new cases appearing during a specified period) and the prevalence (a cross-sectional count of the number of cases at a specified point in time) of pressure ulcers because methodological limitations have prevented researchers from drawing meaningful conclusions from available data. These problems exist in data available from acute care hospitals, long term care facilities, and home care settings. The NPUAP Consensus Development Conference (NPUAP, 1989) broadly categorized the methodological barriers to interpreting the results of incidence and prevalence studies into three problem areas: (1) Study populations were not always comparable (e.g., data collected in tertiary care hospitals are not likely to reflect the findings in community hospitals); (2) sources of data ranged from direct observation of patients by trained research personnel to information retrieved from patient records; and (3) study methods often confused incidence and prevalence data, included ulcers at different stages, or excluded segments of the institutionalized population.

In hospital settings, the incidence of pressure ulcers has ranged from 2.7 percent (Gerson, 1975) to 29.5 percent (Clarke and Kadhom, 1988). Prevalence by hospital bed ranged from 4 percent (Ek and Boman, 1982) to 69 percent (Ameis, Chiarcossi, and Jimenez, 1980), whereas the prevalence by hospitalized patients varied between 3.5 percent (Shannon and Skorga, 1989) and 29.5 percent (Oot-Giromini, Bidwell, Heller, et al., 1989). In the most extensive study of acute care facilities, Meehan (1990) surveyed 148 hospitals and found that the prevalence of pressure ulcers was 9.2 percent.

Several special subpopulations may be at higher risk than the general hospital population for pressure ulcer formation. Richardson and Meyer (1981) reported a prevalence of 60 percent among hospitalized quadriplegic patients, and Versluysen (1986) found an incidence of 66 percent among elderly patients admitted for femoral fracture. Orthopedic patients may also be at high risk because they are often immobilized; patients with fractures appear to be at greater risk than those admitted for elective orthopedic procedures (Versluysen, 1985; Jensen and Juncker, 1987). Although few studies have focused on the critical care population, the 33-percent incidence reported by Bergstrom, Demuth, and Braden (1987) and the 41-percent prevalence reported by Robnett (1986) indicate that this group may also be at high risk.

Among persons in skilled care facilities and nursing homes, the prevalence ranged from 2.4 percent (Petersen and Bittmann, 1971) to 23 percent (Langemo, Olson, Hunter, et al., 1989; Young, 1989). Rates obtained in the few incidence studies in this population fall within a comparable range (Brandeis, Morris, Nash, et al., 1990; Langemo, Olson, Hunter, et al., 1991; Powell, 1989). The highly variable nature of case mix and staffing makes generalization concerning these results particularly difficult. According to Brandeis, Morris, Nash, et al. (1990), the incidence of pressure ulcers increases as the length of stay increases. The prevalence and incidence of pressure ulcers in these facilities deserve closer attention to determine the magnitude and cost of this problem and allow administrators to project the resources needed to increase the effectiveness of patient care.

The prevalence of pressure ulcers among persons cared for in the home with the supervision or assistance of professionals is not completely clear, and thus the magnitude of the problem in this population also requires further investigation. Barbenel, Jordan, Nicol, et al. (1977) reported a prevalence of 8.7 percent of ulcers designated Stage II or worse. In a relatively small sample ($N = 30$), Clarke and Kadhom (1988) reported an incidence of 20 percent in home care patients. A recent 1-year study of 326 home health care patients reported an incidence of 4.3 percent and a prevalence of 12.9 percent (Hentzen, Bergstrom, and Pozehl, 1993).

In summary, the incidence and prevalence of pressure ulcers are sufficiently high to warrant concern, yet it has been difficult to draw definitive conclusions about the nature and magnitude of this problem. Determining these rates has been complicated because many studies were not sufficiently controlled in terms of data acquisition methods and pressure ulcer classification systems. Studies that use large data bases suffer because the data acquisition skills of the observers are not controlled. Results of these studies must be balanced with results of studies involving smaller samples but having technically more accurate data acquisition methods.

To help correct these methodological problems, the staging system recommended by the NPUAP (1989) should be endorsed and used in future studies to allow the data to be compared and interpreted. In addition, a systematic assessment guide detailing the sites of the pressure ulcers should be used to prevent errors of omission in measurement. Information about the incidence and prevalence of pressure ulcers that takes into account the stage of the lesion, the type of health care facility, the specific diagnosis, the individual's level of mobility, and other risk factors will permit administrators to plan and allocate services to those populations at risk for this condition.

Methodology for Guideline Development

The procedures followed for developing this guideline were those recommended by AHCPR and by Steven Woolf, MD, MPH, a consultant to the panel. The procedures were further influenced by consultation with JoAnne Horsley, PhD, RN, FAAN, the principal investigator for the Conduct and Utilization of Research in Nursing (CURN), a pioneering project in research utilization funded during the late 1970's. The CURN project developed practice protocols based on a critique of available research and a synthesis of current knowledge (Haller, Reynolds, and Horsley, 1979).

The panel used the methodology recommended by AHCPR to develop recommendations based on (1) the clinical benefits and harms of potential interventions and (2) relevant health policy issues. Assessment of the former was intended to determine which practices produce the best health outcome for patients in the aggregate sense, and assessment of the latter was intended to address resource constraints (e.g., costs of interventions) and feasibility issues that might affect implementation of the panel's recommendations.

This guideline offers recommendations about how health care professionals can provide quality care. The recommendations are based on current scientific evidence and professional judgment and do not determine whether selected procedures are reimbursable; decisions about reimbursement are made by third-party payers. Furthermore, the recommendations do not specify which professionals should perform which procedures; these decisions are based on professional qualifications and State licensing regulations.

Panel members were appointed by AHCPR based on a broad range of input from professional and health care consumer organizations and individuals. At least one professional organization endorsed each panel member.

Over the course of this guideline's development, a total of 20 individuals served as panel members, with panel positions held at various times by seven physicians (family medicine, dermatology, plastic surgery, surgery–nutrition, gerontology, and physical medicine and rehabilitation), seven nurses (rehabilitation, aging, acute care, enterostomal therapy, wound care, nutrition, health care education, and management), one occupational therapist (rehabilitation), two biomedical engineers (rehabilitation), two basic scientists (wound healing), and one consumer representative. The panel also engaged a number of consultants with expertise in geriatric medicine, wound care research, nutrition, health economics, guideline development methodology, research utilization, clinical algorithm development, infection control, and consumer interests.

Traditionally, guidelines and standards have been based on the best judgments of a panel of experts. However, it is no longer deemed sufficient to rely on such judgments alone without a prior understanding of the scientific data base. Thus, the panel was charged with summarizing the scientific data to support guideline recommendations. The National Library of Medicine (NLM) conducted a comprehensive literature review based on panel requests, and panel members scrutinized evidence of clinical benefits or harms and reviewed prevailing practice as documented in professional standards and written reports. Retrieval of published manuscripts and relevant unpublished material was comprehensive. Relevant literature was identified through computerized searches of articles published between 1966 and May 1, 1993. MEDLARS was the primary data base searched, with supplemental data bases used as necessary. Literature was also identified through (1) hand searches of journals not referenced in computerized data bases; (2) reference lists from review articles; (3) personal files of panelists; (4) recommendations of peer reviewers, open forum participants, and companies manufacturing products used to treat pressure ulcers; and (5) research reports submitted by investigators engaged in pressure ulcer research. Through these mechanisms, the panel reviewed more than 45,000 abstracts (including duplicates from several data bases). About 1,700 manuscripts were selected for further evaluation based on the inclusion criteria established by the panel; 40 percent of these were research manuscripts. All research manuscripts, whether published or unpublished, were evaluated for quality and were included only if they met the quality standards and content-based inclusion criteria established by the panel. Eventually, 333 references were cited to support this guideline.

The guideline was written after the panel evaluated the scientific evidence and expert clinical opinion and considered the benefits and harms of each potential recommendation. Recommendations were based on the quality and quantity of supporting research evidence (either direct or indirect) indicating that a certain action would produce a favorable result. In the absence of conclusive research evidence, expert opinion was sought and documented as such. Expert opinion (as reflected in review articles, textbooks, the standards and guidelines set by professional organizations, and the judgment of panel members and peer reviewers) is an important part of guideline development because it is unlikely that an adequate scientific data base will exist to support every recommendation.

The experience of the CURN project showed that guidelines are most effective when they are specific (Haller, Reynolds, and Horsley, 1979). For this reason, the panel attempted to be as specific as possible while allowing enough flexibility to respect expert judgment and patient preferences in individual cases.

Following completion of an outline of the guideline document, an open forum was announced in the *Federal Register* and was held in Washington, DC, on April 9, 1992. All persons, organizations, and agencies with an interest in the pressure ulcer treatment guideline were invited to attend and to present written or verbal testimony. A draft version of the document was then presented at a conference held on March 5–6, 1993, sponsored by the NPUAP and WOCN and attended by more than 300 persons. This conference enabled all participants to provide feedback on the content and format of the document through formal response and a computer-assisted critique. Conference sessions were also held in which individuals representing acute care, long-term care, and home care settings provided input.

Next, an additional formal peer review was undertaken. Peer reviewers were selected from the following groups:

1. Professional organizations. These organizations were invited to disseminate the guideline to as many reviewers as deemed appropriate and to collate responses in order to submit to the panel a single document containing reviewer comments.

2. Participants in the open forum and NPUAP and WOCN conference as well as other professional participants who volunteered.

3. Government regulatory agencies. Copies of the guideline were sent to the Health Care Financing Administration, the FDA, and the CDC. Several individuals within these agencies served as peer reviewers; however, their review does not constitute official agency review and approval.

4. Interested health care providers and consumers who expressed to the panel chair or panel members their willingness to review the guideline.

A list of potential peer reviewers was maintained throughout the project. Those finally selected represented a broad range of professional disciplines, clinical practice arenas, and geographic regions. Peer review by professional organizations and Government regulatory agencies does not constitute endorsement of the guideline. Peer reviewers were asked specifically to evaluate (1) the comprehensiveness of the literature review and identify any literature evidence that was omitted or inappropriately or incompletely cited, (2) the conclusions based on the literature review and analysis, and (3) the guideline recommendations based on practical realities. Their comments were distributed to panel members, whose subsequent deliberations led to revisions of the guideline.

The panel also subjected the pressure ulcer treatment guideline to pilot review, which comprised three specific activities. First, health care agencies were invited to examine the hypothetical impact of the guideline on their setting in terms of cost, resources, and practicability. Second, health care agencies were invited to examine the guideline, test it informally on a small number of patients in the practice setting, and provide feedback to the panel. Third, selected sites were asked to provide a somewhat more formal evaluation of the guideline, as time allowed, setting in motion a plan for implementing guideline recommendations. Such in-depth testing provided additional useful information prior to final revisions.

Pilot review sites, like peer reviewers, were selected from a list of names submitted to the panel during the process of guideline development. Key organizations representing various classifications of health care settings were asked to conduct pilot reviews. A broad diversity of clinical representation was sought. University, community, and small rural hospitals were selected as well as nursing home chains, small private nursing homes, and visiting-nurse and other home health care agencies. Attention was also given to the geographic distribution of pilot reviewers.

The results of peer and pilot review were collated, and appropriate suggestions were incorporated into the guideline. The revised guideline was then submitted to AHCPR for publication.

Strength-of-Evidence Ratings

The panel assigned each recommendation a rating of A, B, or C to indicate the strength of the evidence supporting the recommendation. The ratings were based on the following criteria:

A Results of two or more randomized controlled clinical trials on pressure ulcers in humans provide support.

B Results of two or more controlled clinical trials on pressure ulcers in humans provide support, or when appropriate, results of two or more controlled trials in an animal model provide indirect support.

C This rating requires one or more of the following: (1) Results of one controlled trial; (2) results of at least two case series/descriptive studies on pressure ulcers in humans; or (3) expert opinion.

This approach was adapted from *Guide to Clinical Preventive Services* by the U.S. Preventive Services Task Force (1989). Evidence ratings are based on the number of studies (quantity), quality of research, number of replications, and consistency of findings.

It is important to clarify that these ratings represent the strength of the supporting research evidence, not the strength of the recommendation itself. The strength of each recommendation is conveyed in the language used to describe it. For example, the panel's directive to "cleanse wounds initially and at each dressing change" leaves little doubt that this measure is strongly recommended as a time-honored, efficacious treatment, despite an evidence rating of C. On the other hand, the recommendation to consider electrical stimulation therapy under certain conditions is less directive, despite stronger supporting research evidence. Although electrical stimulation has been shown to enhance the rate of healing in clinical trials, it is a relatively new technology that has not been used extensively in clinical practice.

Economic Impact and Public Policy Implications

The eventual economic impact of the utilization of the guideline's recommendations is difficult to determine. Miller and Delozier (1994) estimated the baseline costs of pressure ulcer treatment under two scenarios. Although the data bases used by these investigators have limitations such as underreporting of pressure ulcers and approximations of physician fees rather than actual costs, this study provides a reasonably accurate estimate of the costs of pressure ulcers in 1992.

According to this analysis, the mean hospital charge for patients with a primary diagnosis of pressure ulcers was $21,675, and estimated physician charges were $2,900 per case. The total charges for 34,000 inpatients with a primary diagnosis of pressure ulcer were $836 million. To illustrate the costs of pressure ulcers as a secondary diagnosis, hip fracture patients with and without pressure ulcers were compared. An average of $10,986 in additional hospital charges was attributed to the pressure ulcers. When estimated physician fees of $1,200 per case were included, the total cost of pressure ulcers as a complication of hip fracture was $84 million. Although less specific cost data are available for nursing home facilities and home care settings, Miller and Delozier conservatively estimate that the 1992 costs of pressure ulcer care in these settings was $355 million and $60 million, respectively. The total estimated cost for all settings was $1.335 billion.

The economic impact of guideline implementation was estimated by comparing the costs of care recommended by the guideline with the cost of the care that is currently provided. Although in some cases the costs of initial services (e.g., more complete assessments, frequent repositioning, thorough wound cleansing) would increase, these costs are minimal when compared with the costs of the more intensive care required to treat large or recalcitrant pressure ulcers. Guideline implementation should save money by reducing the need for high acuity care, expensive equipment, and special procedures while minimally increasing the funds dedicated to "low tech care" (e.g., provision of adequate personnel to feed and turn patients). Although it is difficult to assess the magnitude of savings, Miller and

Delozier suggest that guideline implementation is likely to save at least $40 million (or 3 percent) of the total costs measured by their analysis.

One policy question raised by this analysis is whether committing more resources to the prevention and initial care of pressure ulcers with the expectation of avoiding the higher human and economic costs of treating more advanced ulcers would be feasible and advantageous. In the interest of ensuring high-quality, cost-effective patient care, this question warrants serious consideration by consumers, care providers, third-party payers, and Government regulatory agencies.

Followup Activities

Recommendations for followup activities should focus on expanded programs of research in this area. Monitoring the incidence and prevalence of pressure ulcers at various stages and in various settings would help in evaluating the impact of the pressure ulcer prevention and treatment guidelines. Such studies should use the standard pressure ulcer classification system recommended in this document. A reliable system to accurately identify Stage I pressure ulcers in individuals with darkly pigmented skin should be developed.

Research is needed regarding the assessment and management of pressure ulcer pain and the relationship between psychosocial status and healing. Continued monitoring of the results of studies in which cytokine growth factors are being used to promote healing, as well as studies on the efficacy of electrical stimulation, would be beneficial. The use of clean rather than sterile dressings warrants further investigation. The panel would also like to see continued investigation of the extent of use and efficacy of various types of support surfaces, both static and dynamic. In addition, multisite controlled clinical trials comparing surgical and medical management of pressure ulcers should be conducted. One important part of such studies should be an analysis of costs.

Ideally, "healing" is the outcome that should be measured in pressure ulcer treatment studies. Studies measuring intermediate outcomes (such as partial healing or a decrease in the size of the ulcer) make more limited contributions to the scientific data base. All treatment studies should carefully describe the "usual care" that is administered to control subjects.

Several programmatic changes were recommended by the panel, such as more extensive formation of quality improvement teams and educational programs and greater use of nutritional assessment instruments and nutritional supplementation. Evaluating the application of these recommendations will advance knowledge in this field.

Organization of the Guideline

This guideline is organized to correspond with the pertinent aspects of pressure ulcer care: Assessing the pressure ulcer and the patient; managing tissue loads; caring for the ulcer; managing bacterial colonization and infection; repairing ulcers surgically; providing education for patients, families, and caregivers; and improving the quality of care through quality improvement programs. The guideline reflects the state of current knowledge, as contained in the health care literature, regarding the effectiveness and appropriateness of procedures and practices designed to treat pressure ulcers. In the *Clinical Practice Guideline*, the panel provides recommendations for the treatment of pressure ulcers along with a synopsis of evidence supporting each recommendation. The guideline recommendations alone, without the supporting evidence, can be found in the *Quick Reference Guide for Clinicians*. A more complete discussion of relevant research as well as tables summarizing the evidence appears in the full *Guideline Technical Report*. Finally, a *Consumer Version* is available in English and Spanish.

Clinical Algorithm

The overview algorithm in Figure 1 provides the clinician with a visual display of the conceptual organization, procedural flow, decision points, and preferred management pathways discussed in the guideline. When applied to individual patients, this algorithm should be adapted to accommodate patient preferences and overall patient goals. Numbers in the algorithm correspond to the explanations that follow it. Subalgorithms that expand on nutritional assessment and support, management of tissue loads, ulcer care, and management of infection have been incorporated within the relevant chapters of this document. The various shapes in all algorithms have the following meanings: (1) Diamonds designate "yes-no" decisions; (2) rectangles designate interventions; (3) hexagons designate the need for patient education and counseling; and (4) ovals refer the reader to previous nodes in the algorithm.

1. **Pressure Ulcer Identification.** The pressure ulcer treatment guideline provides recommendations concerning the evaluation and management of patients with established Stage II, III, and IV pressure ulcers. A separate guideline *(Pressure Ulcers in Adults: Prediction and Prevention. Clinical Practice Guideline, No. 3)* describes strategies for identifying high-risk patients, preventing ulcers, and treating Stage I pressure ulcers.

2. **Initial Assessment.** The initial assessment of patients with pressure ulcers has several dimensions: (a) Assessment of the pressure ulcer, (b) complete history and physical examination, (c) assessment for complications and comorbidities, (d) nutritional status assessment,

Figure 1. Management of pressure ulcers: overview

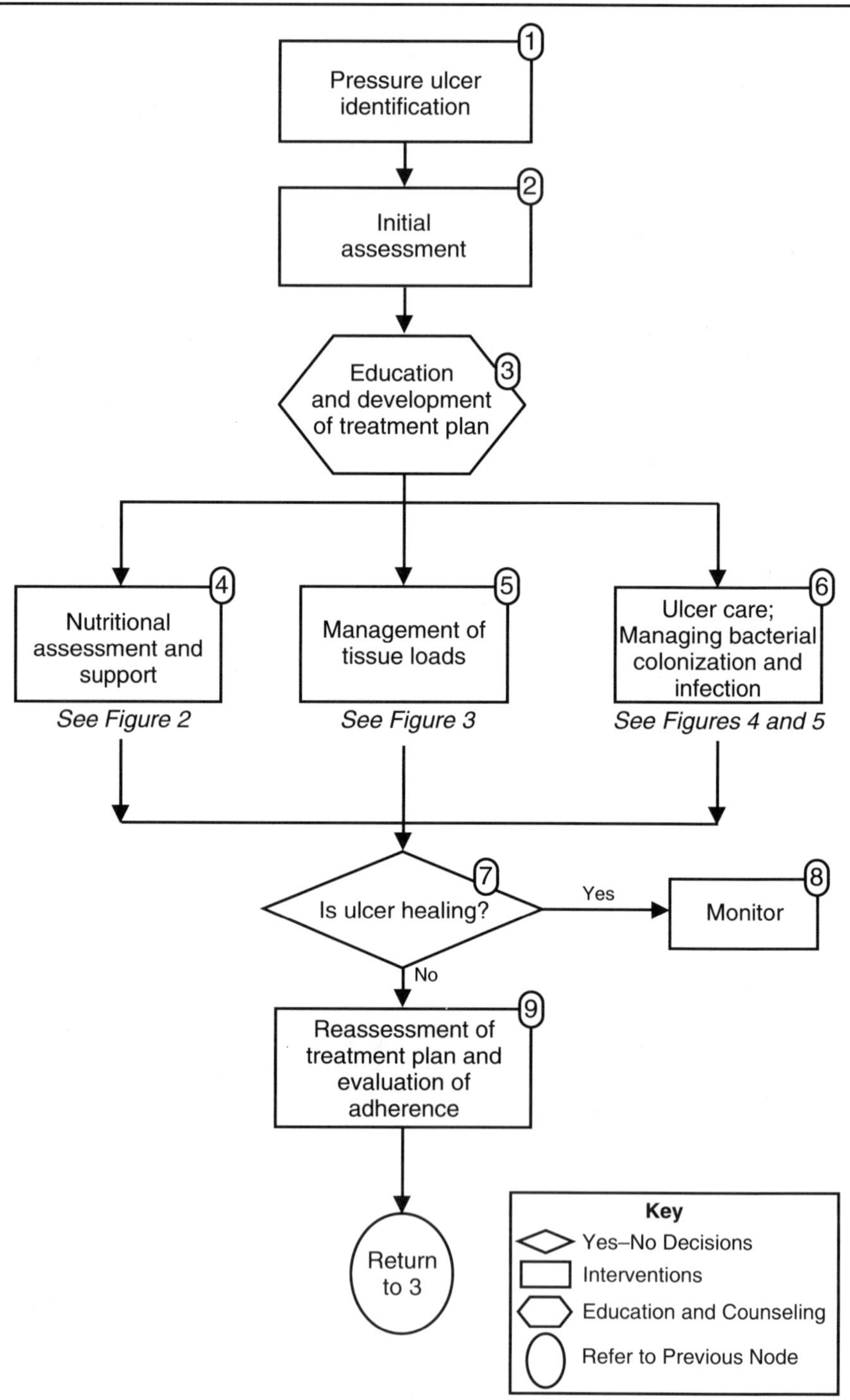

(e) pain assessment, (f) psychosocial evaluation, and (g) assessment of risk for developing additional pressure ulcers.

An assessment of the pressure ulcer should determine the location, stage, size, and depth of the wound, as well as the presence or absence of sinus tracts, undermining, tunneling, exudate, necrotic tissue, epithelialization, and granulation tissue. The history and physical examination should address concurrent illnesses and conditions that might affect wound healing, including nutritional deficits and neurological, vascular, endocrine, or immunological abnormalities. The psychosocial evaluation should focus on the patient's cognitive capacities and ability to help develop and adhere to treatment plans. The extent of social support should be assessed, with arrangements made to provide assistance with home care if needed. In addition, the degree of pain produced by the ulcer should be evaluated and appropriate steps taken to minimize any pain or discomfort. (Readers are referred to the AHCPR-sponsored guideline, *Acute Pain Management: Operative or Medical Procedures and Trauma. Clinical Practice Guideline, No. 1.)* Patients judged to be at high risk for additional pressure ulcers should be identified and appropriate precautions taken. (Refer to *Pressure Ulcers in Adults: Prediction and Prevention. Clinical Practice Guideline, No. 3.*)

3. **Education and Development of Treatment Plan.** After the initial assessment is completed, patients and family caregivers should be provided with information sufficient to enable them to understand the treatment of pressure ulcers and assist in developing a treatment plan.

   The treatment plan should reflect the patient's values and explicitly define the goals of therapy. In general, the primary goal is healing of the ulcer, but sometimes the goal of patient comfort may take precedence. An example might be the patient with a terminal medical condition who experiences pain or agitation on turning or during administration of tube feedings (to correct malnutrition); another patient may simply wish to forgo the sort of intensive management that may be required to heal advanced pressure ulcers. Although the recommendations in this guideline apply primarily to patients for whom the goal of therapy is wound healing, they are also applicable, in whole or in part, to patients seeking palliative care.

   An effective pressure ulcer treatment plan should have three components: (a) Nutritional assessment and support, (b) management of tissue loads, and (c) ulcer care and management of bacterial colonization and infection. These three treatment components are equally important and essential aspects of pressure ulcer management. As can be seen in the algorithm in Figure 1, these three issues should be addressed simultaneously.

4. **Nutritional Assessment and Support.** (See Figure 2 in Chapter 2, Assessment.) Nutritional assessment is essential for identifying individuals whose nutritional status may compromise healing. Assessment also serves as a basis for planning nutritional support.

5. **Management of Tissue Loads.** (See Figure 3 in Chapter 3, Managing Tissue Loads.) Management of tissue loads (i.e., pressure, friction, and shear) is a critical component of any pressure ulcer treatment plan.

6. **Ulcer Care.** (See Figure 4 in Chapter 4, Ulcer Care, and Figure 5 in Chapter 5, Managing Bacterial Colonization and Infection.) Care of the pressure ulcer involves debridement, wound cleansing, the application of dressings, and measures to control bacterial colonization and treat infection.

7. **Assessment of Ulcer Healing.** Progress toward healing should be evaluated at least weekly. If signs of ulcer deterioration are observed sooner (e.g., during daily dressing changes), steps to reverse them should be taken immediately. If the patient's general condition deteriorates (e.g., signs of sepsis), the ulcer should be reassessed promptly. Healing should be evaluated using the same criteria discussed under initial assessment (Node 2), that is, size, depth, and the presence of exudate, epithelialization, granulation tissue, and findings such as necrotic tissue, sinus tracts, undermining, tunneling, and purulent drainage or other signs of infection. A clean pressure ulcer with adequate innervation and blood supply should show progress toward healing in 2 to 4 weeks.

8. **Monitoring.** Healing ulcers should be assessed regularly to ensure continued progress toward the goal of complete healing. Caregivers should continue to monitor the individual's general health, nutritional adequacy, psychosocial support, and pain level and should be alert to signs of complications (e.g., advancing cellulitis, sinus tract or abscess, meningitis, endocarditis, septic arthritis, osteomyelitis, sepsis). The frequency of monitoring should be determined by the clinician based on the condition of the patient, the condition of the ulcer, the rate of healing, and the type of health care setting.

9. **Reassessment of Treatment Plan and Evaluation of Adherence.** If the ulcer is not healing, the clinician must reassess the treatment plan and determine whether it is being followed. If necessary, the plan and strategies for its implementation should be revised. In particular, the clinician should assess whether tissue load management is adequate and should evaluate the extent of adherence to cleansing, dressing, and nutritional support interventions. Necrotic tissue or underlying abscesses should be suspected if the ulcer is not healing, and if found, removed or drained. Evaluation and treatment of pressure ulcer infection and underlying osteomyelitis should also be undertaken.

2 Assessment

Assessment is the starting point in preparing to treat or manage an individual with a pressure ulcer. Assessment involves the entire person, not just the ulcer, and is the basis for planning treatment and evaluating its effects. Adequate assessment is also essential for communication among caregivers. This chapter provides recommendations for assessing both the pressure ulcer and the individual. Assessment of the individual addresses physical health, common complications, nutritional status, pain level, and psychosocial health.

Assessing the Pressure Ulcer

Assess the pressure ulcer(s) initially for location, stage (NPUAP, 1989), size, sinus tracts, undermining, tunneling, exudate, necrotic tissue, and the presence or absence of granulation tissue and epithelialization. (See Attachment A for a sample pressure ulcer assessment guide.) (Strength of Evidence = C.)

Pressure ulcers should be uniformly described to facilitate communication among staff and to ensure adequate monitoring of the progress toward healing. The system developed by the National Pressure Ulcer Advisory Panel (NPUAP, 1989) is a synthesis of the most commonly used staging methods. Necrotic tissue must be removed before the stage of the ulcer can be determined. To monitor progress or deterioration of the lesion, the examiner must accurately measure the length, width, and depth of the ulcer and describe sinus tracts, tunneling, undermining, necrotic tissue, exudate, and the presence or absence of granulation tissue and epithelialization (Yarkony, Kirk, Carlson, et al., 1990). Color photographs, taken on initial assessment and reevaluation, are very helpful in monitoring ulcer healing.

Reassess pressure ulcers at least weekly (as shown in Attachment A). If the condition of the patient or of the wound deteriorates, reevaluate the treatment plan as soon as any evidence of deterioration is noted. (Strength of Evidence = C.)

To determine the adequacy of the treatment plan, it is essential to monitor pressure ulcers at consistent intervals. Assessment and documentation should be carried out at least weekly, unless there is evidence of deterioration, in which case both the pressure ulcer and the patient's overall management must be reassessed immediately. In the home setting, this may require the assistance of the patient and family, because weekly assessment by health care providers is not always feasible.

Indicators of a deteriorating pressure ulcer include increases in exudate and wound edema, loss of granulation tissue, and a purulent discharge. The onset of impaired mental status, fever, hypotension, and tachycardia may indicate sudden deterioration of the patient's physical status.

A comprehensive literature review failed to identify one tool for reassessment and monitoring that could be recommended. The suggested assessment guide is based on the work of Bates-Jensen (1990) and numerous other investigators; with further research, the Bates-Jensen scale may prove useful for monitoring and reassessment. However, to date, no one tool for reassessment and monitoring can be recommended.

A clean pressure ulcer should show evidence of some healing within 2 to 4 weeks. If no progress can be demonstrated, reevaluate the adequacy of the overall treatment plan as well as adherence to this plan, making modifications as necessary. (Strength of Evidence = C.)

A pressure ulcer with adequate innervation and vascular supply should show evidence of healing within 2 to 4 weeks (Robson, Phillips, Thomason, et al., 1992a, 1992b; van Rijswijk, 1993). Suboptimal healing may be attributed to inadequacies of the treatment plan or failure to adhere to the treatment plan (e.g., failure to alleviate the pressure, to apply proper dressings, or to correct nutritional deficiencies). These contributing factors can be influenced by psychosocial or economic variables. Although healing is always the preferred goal, maintenance of comfort may be an appropriate goal for a terminally ill patient.

Assessing the Individual With a Pressure Ulcer

History and Physical Examination

Perform a complete history and physical examination, because a pressure ulcer should be assessed in the context of the patient's overall physical and psychosocial health. (Strength of Evidence = C.)

Efforts to ensure good health require a thorough understanding of the individual patient's overall physical and mental status regardless of the specific illness being treated. In the case of pressure ulcers, the individual's capacity to heal may be limited by comorbid illnesses such as peripheral vascular disease, diabetes mellitus, immune deficiencies, collagen vascular diseases, malignancies, psychosis, and depression (Lazarus, Cooper, Knighton, et al., 1992).

Assessing Complications

Clinicians should be alert to the potential complications associated with pressure ulcers. (Strength of Evidence = C.)

The following complications are associated with pressure ulcers:

- Amyloidosis (Melcher, Longe, and Gelbart, 1988).

- Endocarditis (Schwartz and Pervez, 1971).
- Heterotopic bone formation (Reuler and Cooney, 1981).
- Maggot infestation (Roche, Cross, Burgess, et al., 1990).
- Meningitis (Soriano, Aguado, Tornero, et al., 1986).
- Perineal–urethral fistula (Hackler and Zampieri, 1987).
- Pseudoaneurysm (Wang, Lineaweaver, Scott, et al., 1987).
- Septic arthritis (Klein, Moore, Capen, et al., 1988).
- Sinus tract or abscess (Putnam, Calenoff, Betts, et al., 1978).
- Squamous cell carcinoma in the ulcer (Berkwits, Yarkony, and Lewis, 1986).
- Systemic complications of topical treatment—e.g., iodine toxicity (Shetty and Duthie, 1990) and hearing loss after topical neomycin and systemic gentamicin (Johnson, 1988).

Three other complications—osteomyelitis, bacteremia, and advancing cellulitis—are discussed in Chapter 5, Managing Bacterial Colonization and Infection.

The clinician who is treating a patient with a pressure ulcer must be aware of the numerous possible complications of pressure ulcers that have been reported in the literature. Some complications are infectious, such as abscess, sinus tract, meningitis, and endocarditis, and others are noninfectious. Even a relatively small opening in the skin can connect with an extensive cavity or with a deeply penetrating sinus tract. Computerized tomography (CT) scanning was reported to be effective in detecting deep abscesses associated with pressure ulcers (Firooznia, Rafii, Golimbu, et al., 1983a, 1983b). Sinography was reported to be useful for defining the extent of sinus tracts underlying pressure ulcers (Hooker, Sibley, Nemchausky, et al., 1988; Putnam, Calenoff, Betts, et al., 1978). The clinician must also be aware that some treatments of pressure ulcers may lead to other complications. For example, topical treatment with iodine-containing agents may unmask subclinical hyperthyroidism (Shetty and Duthie, 1990) or result in iodine toxicity (Aronoff, Friedman, Doedens, et al., 1980). Topical aminoglycoside treatment has been associated with hearing loss (Johnson, 1988).

Nutritional Assessment and Management

Because many studies have linked pressure ulcers with malnutrition, screening for nutritional deficiencies is an important part of the initial assessment. The goal of nutritional assessment and management is to ensure that the diet of the individual with a pressure ulcer contains nutrients adequate to support healing. The following recommendations and the algorithm depicted in Figure 2 are designed to guide the clinician in meeting this goal.

Figure 2. Nutritional assessment and support

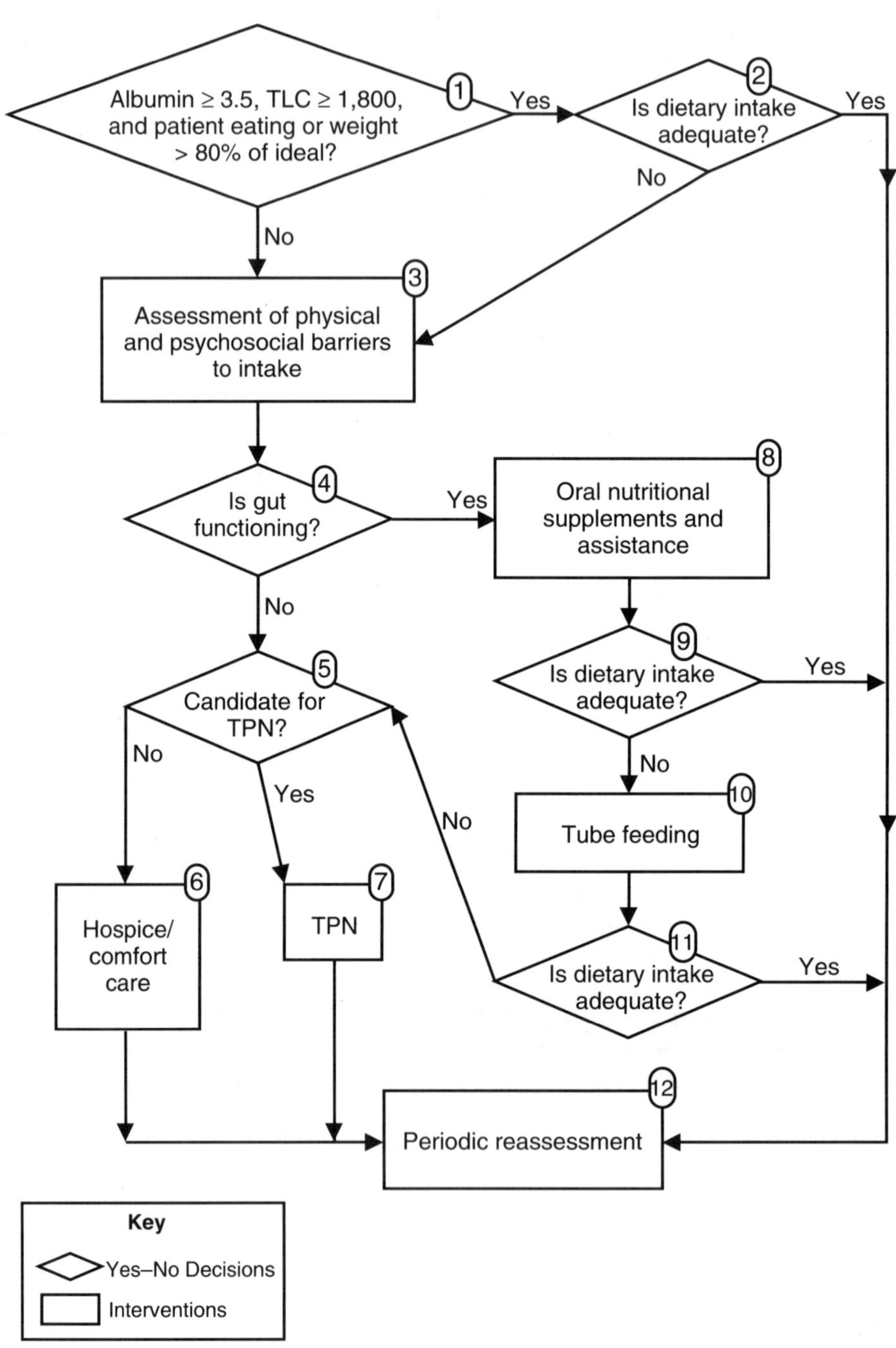

Note: TLC = total lymphocyte count; TPN = total parenteral nutrition.

Ensure adequate dietary intake to prevent malnutrition to the extent that this is compatible with the individual's wishes. (Strength of Evidence = B.)

Multiple studies indicate that malnutrition is a risk factor for pressure ulcer formation. Furthermore, the stage of the wound is correlated with the severity of nutritional deficits, particularly low protein intake or a below-normal serum albumin (Allman, Laprade, Noel, et al., 1986; Bergstrom and Braden, 1992; Berlowitz and Wilking, 1989; Breslow, Hallfrisch, and Goldberg, 1991; Ek, Unosson, and Bjurulf, 1989; Hanan and Scheele, 1991; Holmes, Macchiano, Jhangiani, et al., 1987; Pinchcofsky-Devin and Kaminski, 1986). Prevention of malnutrition will reduce an individual's risk for ulcer formation.

Perform an abbreviated nutritional assessment, as defined by the Nutrition Screening Initiative, at least every 3 months for individuals at risk for malnutrition. These include individuals who are unable to take food by mouth or who experience an involuntary change in weight. (Strength of Evidence = C.)

In patients at risk for malnutrition, an involuntary increase or decrease in weight of 5 percent is predictive of a drop in serum albumin (*Nutrition Screening Manual for Professionals Caring for Older Americans: Nutrition Screening Initiative*, 1991). Because the state of hydration affects weight and albumin concentration, it should also be part of a nutritional screening assessment. (Attachment B is a sample assessment guide.) Clinically significant malnutrition is diagnosed if (1) serum albumin is less than 3.5 mg/dL, (2) total lymphocyte count is less than 1,800/mm^3, or (3) body weight has decreased more than 15 percent. Oral and cutaneous signs of vitamin or mineral deficiencies should also be considered during the nutritional assessment. (Attachment C lists these signs.)

Encourage dietary intake or supplementation if an individual with a pressure ulcer is malnourished. If dietary intake continues to be inadequate, impractical, or impossible, nutritional support (usually tube feeding) should be used to place the patient into positive nitrogen balance (approximately 30 to 35 calories/kg/day and 1.25 to 1.50 grams of protein/kg/day) according to the goals of care. (Strength of Evidence = C.)

A review of the literature suggests that a pressure ulcer can be a grave indicator of malnutrition. Breslow, Hallfrisch, Guy, et al. (1993) found that high-protein diets with increased caloric contents may enhance pressure ulcer healing in malnourished nursing home patients. When the nutritional assessment confirms that the individual is malnourished, the first intervention consists of assisted oral feeding and oral supplements. A second assessment should be done within 3 working days to determine whether intake goals have been achieved. If intake is still inadequate, tube feeding should be initiated to achieve a positive nitrogen balance.

Tests to assess nitrogen balance may not be practical in all settings. For most patients, however, positive nitrogen balance is usually accomplished when intake reaches 30 to 35 calories/kg/day and 1.25 to 1.50 grams of protein/kg/day (Chernoff, Milton, and Lipschitz, 1990; Kaminski, 1976), although as much as 2.00 grams of protein/kg/day may be needed Mulholland, Tui, Wright, et al., 1943). Several reports showed that the presence of a feeding tube in a patient with a pressure ulcer does not necessarily mean that he or she is receiving adequate support (*Nutrition Screening Manual for Professionals Caring for Older Americans: Nutrition Screening Initiative*, 1991). Repeat nutritional assessments, including measurements of serial protein markers such as serum albumin, should be used to evaluate nutritional support. Monitoring for safety and tolerance, including the possibility of loose bowel movements related to tube feedings, should also be ongoing. (Attachment D outlines the steps in the practical management of loose bowel movements in tube-fed patients.)

Give vitamin and mineral supplements if deficiencies are confirmed or suspected. (Strength of Evidence = C.)

Vitamin and mineral deficiencies have been demonstrated in the majority of patients in nursing home studies (Bergstrom and Braden, 1992; Pinchcofsky-Devin and Kaminski, 1986). There is some evidence that vitamin C and zinc supplementation may aid healing in the presence of deficiencies (Burr, 1973; Taylor, Rimmer, Day, et al., 1974). (Attachment C identifies possible oral and cutaneous signs of vitamin deficiencies.) A daily high-potency vitamin and mineral supplement is recommended for all patients suspected of having vitamin deficiencies. When specific deficiencies are diagnosed, individual supplements of up to 10 times the Recommended Daily Allowance (RDA) for water-soluble vitamins may have to be added to the patient's daily dietary intake (Chen and Fan-Chiang, 1981; Cruz Santiago, Kaminski, and Palencia Salinas, 1981; Williams, Lines, and McKay, 1988).

Pain Assessment and Management

The goal of pain management in the pressure ulcer patient is to eliminate the cause of the pain, to provide analgesia, or both. Additional information regarding pain assessment and management is provided in *Acute Pain Management: Operative or Medical Procedures and Trauma. Clinical Practice Guideline, No. 1.*

Assess all patients for pain related to the pressure ulcer or its treatment. (Strength of Evidence = C.)

Even though the literature on the subject of pain is considerable, including assessment and management (both in general and related to particular sites and causes), there is only cursory mention of pressure ulcer pain. Clinicians report anecdotally that they observe patients reacting to pressure ulcer–related pain during turning, dressing changes, and debridement (Black and Black, 1987; Tudhope, 1984); however, considerable research is needed in this area. Meanwhile, the clinician should recognize that such pain may exist and should assess for its presence. Assessment tools can be found in the acute pain management guideline. Caregivers should not assume because a patient cannot express or respond to pain that it does not exist. Because pain may be evoked or may be especially acute during dressing changes and debridement, the caregiver should try to prevent such discomfort or take steps to relieve it (Acute Pain Management Guideline Panel, 1992).

Manage pain by eliminating or controlling the source of pain (e.g., covering wounds, adjusting support surfaces, repositioning). Provide analgesia as needed and appropriate. (Strength of Evidence = C.)

Management of pressure ulcer–associated pain may require several simultaneous interventions. For example, a combination of repositioning, covering a wound, and systemic analgesia may be needed to relieve pain. The effectiveness of the intervention should be evaluated, with adjustments based on the patient's verbal and physiological responses (Acute Pain Management Guideline Panel, 1992). Research needs to be conducted to determine the most effective pain management techniques for pressure ulcer pain.

Psychosocial Assessment and Management

The goal of a psychosocial assessment is to gather the information necessary to formulate a plan of care consistent with individual and family preferences, goals, and abilities. The goal of psychosocial management is to create an environment conducive to patient adherence to the pressure ulcer treatment plan.

All individuals being treated for pressure ulcers should undergo a psychosocial assessment to determine their ability and motivation to comprehend and adhere to the treatment program. The assessment should include but not be limited to the following:

- **Mental status, learning ability, depression.**
- **Social support.**
- **Polypharmacy or overmedication.**
- **Alcohol and/or drug abuse.**

- **Goals, values, and lifestyle.**
- **Sexuality.**
- **Culture and ethnicity.**
- **Stressors.**

Periodic reassessment is recommended. (Strength of Evidence = C).

This recommendation is based primarily on expert clinical opinion, because little direct research evidence links psychosocial variables with the management of pressure ulcers. There is evidence that mean depression scores are higher among spinal cord–injured individuals who are at high risk for pressure ulcers (Fuhrer, Rintala, Hart, et al., 1993). Knowledge, compliance with treatment, and quality of participation in group psychosocial intervention sessions are reported to be associated with healing (LaMantia, Hirschwald, Goodman, et al., 1987). Other psychosocial variables shown to be related to the incidence of pressure ulcers may also be associated with healing. For example, satisfaction with life activities and responsibility for skin care were associated with a lower incidence of pressure ulcers (Anderson and Andberg, 1979), and alcoholism was associated with a higher incidence of pressure ulcers (Vidal and Sarrias, 1991). Psychosocial counseling and education regarding self-care were found to be associated with positive outcomes related to pressure ulcers (Krouskop, Noble, Garber, et al., 1983).

Assess resources (e.g., availability and skill of caregivers, finances, equipment) of individuals being treated for pressure ulcers in the home. (Strength of Evidence = C.)

This recommendation is based on expert clinical opinion. A successful treatment program in the home requires adequate caregiver and equipment resources (Hentz, 1979). Caregivers need to be evaluated for their ability to comprehend and implement the treatment requirements. Caregivers should also be evaluated for their level of strength and endurance. Economic factors should be considered, because they may limit the supply and availability of equipment as well as opportunities to relieve caregivers.

Set treatment goals consistent with the values and lifestyle of the individual, family, and caregiver. (Strength of Evidence = C.)

This recommendation is based on expert clinical opinion. The clinician should collaborate with the individual and the family in setting treatment goals and should provide opportunities to make adjustments in the treatment plan based on specific needs and preferences of the individual, family, and other caregivers.

Arrange interventions to meet identified psychosocial needs and goals. Followup should be planned in cooperation with the individual and caregiver. (Strength of Evidence = C.)

This recommendation is based on expert clinical opinion. If any of the variables in the psychosocial assessment is found to influence adherence with treatment, efforts should be made—with input from the individual and family members—to alter the situation to enhance effectiveness of treatment. Psychological counseling and education reduced the recurrence of pressure ulcers among patients with spinal cord injuries who were living in the community (Krouskop, Noble, Garber, et al., 1983).

3 Managing Tissue Loads

The goal of the following recommendations is to create an environment that enhances soft tissue viability and promotes healing of the pressure ulcer(s). The term "tissue load" refers to the distribution of pressure, friction, and shear on the tissue. The interventions are designed to decrease the magnitude of tissue loads and to provide levels of moisture and temperature that support tissue health and growth. The algorithm in Figure 3 will help guide clinical decisions on the management of tissue loads.

While in Bed

Positioning techniques and support surfaces for patients in bed are important factors in the management of tissue loads.

Positioning Techniques

Avoid positioning patients on a pressure ulcer. (Strength of Evidence = C.)

Because pressure that is of sufficient intensity and duration to cause soft tissue ischemia and necrosis contributes to the development of pressure ulcers (Kosiak, 1959), it is reasonable to assume that pressure on an ulcer can delay healing.

Use positioning devices to raise a pressure ulcer off the support surface. If the patient is no longer at risk for developing pressure ulcers, these devices may reduce the need for pressure-reducing overlays, mattresses, and beds. Avoid using donut-type devices. (Strength of Evidence = C.)

If a pressure ulcer involves a circumscribed area such as the heel or the back of the head and if the patient is able to reposition the rest of his or her body independently, then using positioning devices to raise the involved area off the support surface may be adequate for healing.

Although ring cushions (donuts) are known to cause venous congestion and edema, few studies have documented their deleterious effects. Crewe (1987), in a study of at-risk patients, found that ring cushions are more likely to cause pressure ulcers than to prevent them.

Establish a written repositioning schedule. (Strength of Evidence = C.)

The schedule for repositioning the patient should be designed to protect uninvolved areas. It should be based on the degree to which the individual is at risk for developing additional pressure ulcers and on the response of the tissue to pressure. Thus, the higher the risk for additional pressure ulcers and the longer the duration of reactive hyperemia, the more frequent-

Figure 3. Management of tissue loads

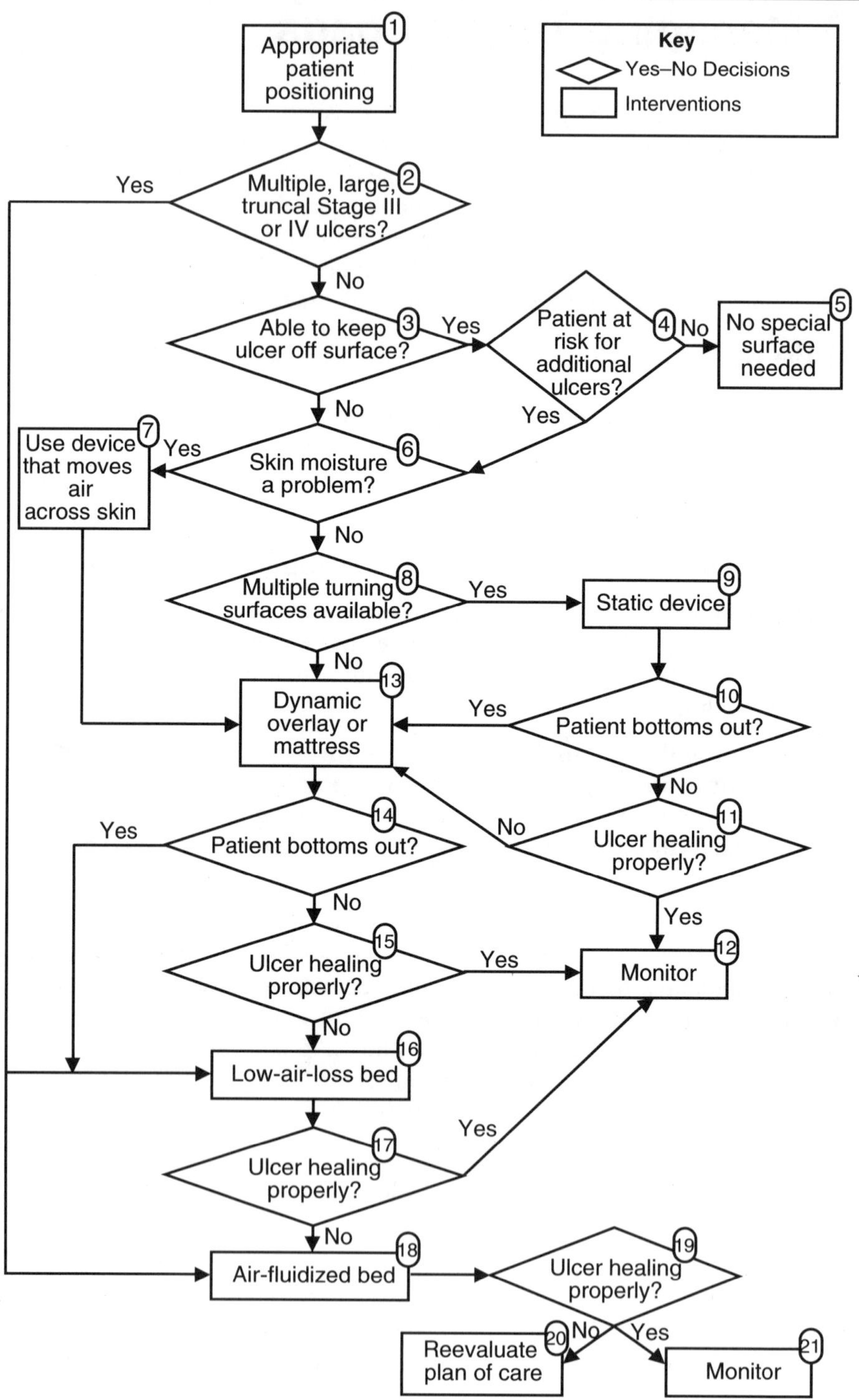

ly the patient should be repositioned.

When the number of pressure ulcers, the patient's condition, or the overall treatment goals make it impossible to avoid positioning a patient on a pressure ulcer, the clinician who is designing the repositioning schedule should keep in mind the need to decrease the duration of pressure on these areas.

Written repositioning schedules should be developed even when patients are using a pressure-reducing support surface. There are numerous reports that patients develop pressure ulcers while using pressure-reducing support surfaces, regardless of the type of surface (Allman, Walker, Hart, et al., 1987; Conine, Daechsel, and Lau, 1990; Jackson, Chagares, Nee, et al., 1988; Parish and Witkowski, 1980; St. Clair, 1992). These surfaces serve only as adjuncts to strategies for positioning and careful monitoring of at-risk patients.

Assess all patients with existing pressure ulcers to determine their risk for developing additional pressure ulcers. For those individuals who remain at risk, institute the following measures recommended in *Pressure Ulcers in Adults: Prediction and Prevention. Clinical Practice Guideline, No. 3:*

- **Avoid positioning immobile individuals directly on their trochanters and use devices such as pillows and foam wedges that totally relieve pressure on the heels, most commonly by raising the heels off the bed. (Strength of Evidence = C.)**

  Redistributing pressure under the heels and over the trochanters is difficult because of the small surface area. Investigators who have measured interface pressure between these areas and support surfaces consistently report high pressures.

- **Use positioning devices such as pillows or foam to prevent direct contact between bony prominences (such as knees or ankles). (Strength of Evidence = C.)**

  This recommendation is based on the usual practice and standards developed by professional organizations.

- **Maintain the head of the bed at the lowest degree of elevation consistent with medical conditions and other restrictions. Limit the amount of time the head of the bed is elevated. (Strength of Evidence = C.)**

  Shearing forces are produced when adjacent surfaces slide across one another. Shear is exerted on the body when the head of the bed is elevated. In this position, the skin and superficial fascia remain fixed against the bed linens while the deep fascia and skeleton slide down toward the foot of the bed. Shear forces are also generated when individuals sitting in a chair slide down in the chair. As a result of shear, blood vessels in the sacral area are likely to become twisted and distorted, and tissue may become ischemic and necrotic (Reichel, 1958). It has been suggested that shear forces contribute to the undermining seen in some sacral ulcers. Standards of professional organizations and clinical articles advocate the use of positioning techniques and devices to help individuals maintain their position in bed or chair.

Support Surfaces

When one is selecting a support surface for a patient, the primary concern should be the therapeutic benefit associated with the product. A variety of support surfaces has been shown to provide an environment in which pressure ulcers improve, but there is no compelling evidence that one support surface consistently performs better than all others, under all circumstances (Allman, Walker, Hart, et al., 1987; Conine, Daechsel, and Lau, 1990; Ferrell, Osterweil, and Christenson, 1993; Jackson, Chagares, Nee, et al., 1986, 1988; Munro, Brown, and Heitman, 1989; Strauss, Gong, Gary, et al., 1991; Warner, 1992; Wiersema and Lueckenotte, 1992). Therefore, the caregiver should consider a variety of factors when selecting a support surface, including the clinical condition of the patient, the characteristics of the care setting, and the characteristics of the support surface.

Table 1 categorizes the various classes of support surfaces according to their performance in counteracting the different forces that contribute to the development of pressure ulcers. After determining which of these forces might be increasing an individual's risk for pressure ulcers, the caregiver may find this table useful in selecting a support surface for a particular

Table 1. Selected characteristics for classes of support surfaces

Performance Characteristics	Support Devices					
	Air-Fluidized	Low-Air-Loss	Alternating Air	Static Flotation (air or water)	Foam	Standard Mattress
Increased support area	Yes	Yes	Yes	Yes	Yes	No
Low moisture retention	Yes	Yes	No	No	No	No
Reduced heat accumulation	Yes	Yes	No	No	No	No
Shear reduction	Yes	?	Yes	Yes	No	No
Pressure reduction	Yes	Yes	Yes	Yes	Yes	No
Dynamic	Yes	Yes	Yes	No	No	No
Cost per day	High	High	Moderate	Low	Low	Low

patient. In addition to considering the features listed in Table 1, caregivers also need to consider other performance factors, such as ease of use, requirements for maintenance, cost, and patient preference (Conine, Choi, and Lim, 1989; Doughty, Fairchild, and Stogis, 1990).

It is important to remember that support surfaces are only one component of a comprehensive treatment plan. If an ulcer does not heal, the entire plan should be reevaluated before the support surface is changed.

Assess all patients with existing pressure ulcers to determine their risk for developing additional pressure ulcers. If the patient remains at risk, use a pressure-reducing surface. (Strength of Evidence = C.)

Patients with existing pressure ulcers may still be at risk for additional pressure ulcers and may therefore need the protection provided by a pressure-reducing surface.

Use a static support surface if a patient can assume a variety of positions without bearing weight on a pressure ulcer and without "bottoming out." (Strength of Evidence = B.)

Although pressure ulcers have been shown to heal when a static support surface is used (Conine, Daechsel, and Lau, 1990; Ferrell, Osterweil, and Christenson, 1993; Warner, 1992; Wiersema and Lueckenotte, 1992), there is no evidence that one type of static support surface is more effective than another. No statistically significant difference in pressure ulcer outcomes has been demonstrated among the available static support surfaces, and thus choice of the static support surface is left to the caregiver. When selecting a static support surface made of foam, caregivers should consider the following characteristics of the foam: stiffness, density, and thickness. Indentation load deflection (ILD) is a measure of stiffness. Typical values for foam mattress overlays would be a 25-percent ILD of 30 pounds, a density of 1.3 pounds per cubic foot, and a thickness of 3 to 4 inches (Kemp and Krouskop, 1994).

The phenomenon of "bottoming out" can be a problem when a mattress overlay is used. The caregiver can determine whether the patient has bottomed out by placing an outstretched hand (palm up) under the overlay below the pressure ulcer or below the part of the body at risk for a pressure ulcer. If the caregiver feels less than an inch of support material, the patient has bottomed out. Bottoming out should be checked at various anatomical sites and while the patient assumes various body positions. For example, when the patient is supine, check for bottoming out at the sacrum and heels. When the patient is side lying, check at the trochanter. When the patient is sitting, check at the ischial tuberosities.

Use a dynamic support surface if the patient cannot assume a variety of positions without bearing weight on a pressure ulcer, if the patient fully compresses the static support surface, or if the pressure ulcer does not

show evidence of healing. (Strength of Evidence = B.)

Although some patients with pressure ulcers improve when cared for on a static support surface, there is evidence that others have a better pressure ulcer outcome when cared for on a dynamic support surface (Ferrell, Osterweil, and Christenson, 1993). The dynamic support surface should be dependable and capable of lifting the individual and preventing bottoming out.

If a patient has large Stage III or Stage IV pressure ulcers on multiple turning surfaces, a low-air-loss bed or an air-fluidized bed may be indicated. (Strength of Evidence = C.)

There is some evidence that patients in the acute care setting who have large pressure ulcers may benefit from the use of an air-fluidized bed (Allman, Walker, Hart, et al., 1987). Several groups have developed criteria for selecting pressure-reducing support surfaces and have targeted patients with Stage III and Stage IV pressure ulcers for treatment on air-fluidized beds (National Center for Cost Containment, 1992; Nimit, 1989; University Hospital Consortium, 1990). Although air-fluidized beds may benefit some patients, these beds are very heavy, and not all structures can accommodate them. Furthermore, transferring patients in and out of air-fluidized beds is difficult (Allman, Walker, Hart, et al., 1987; Smoot, 1986), and adverse side effects (e.g., corneal abrasion from loose beads) have been reported (Smoot, 1986). These drawbacks should be considered before one chooses this type of support surface. Additional studies of air-fluidized bed therapy are needed, particularly in long-term care settings.

Four randomized controlled trials of low-air-loss beds involving a total of 259 subjects with pressure ulcers were reviewed (Ferrell, Osterweil, and Christenson, 1993; Mulder and Seeley, 1991; Warner, 1992; Wiersema and Lueckenotte, 1992). The healing and improvement rates for low-air-loss therapy ranged from 64 to 80 percent in these four studies, and the control therapies showed rates ranging from 47 to 68 percent. One trial involving 84 nursing home residents showed that healing occurred 2.5 times faster among subjects on low-air-loss beds than among those on foam mattresses —a statistically significant difference (Ferrell, Osterweil, and Christenson, 1993). The other three trials were performed in acute care hospitals, and differences in wound healing outcomes for patients on low-air-loss beds versus control treatments did not reach statistical significance in these studies. This may be due to the real absence of clinically important differences in outcome or to characteristics of the research design and implementation (such as inadequate sample sizes or the shorter length of followup possible in acute care settings). Determining the effectiveness of low-air-loss beds definitively will require larger studies with longer followup periods, particularly in the acute care hospital setting.

No studies have compared the effectiveness of low-air-loss beds and air-fluidized beds. Unlike air-fluidized beds, low-air-loss beds can be raised and lowered, and the heads of these beds can be elevated. In addition, transferring patients in or out of bed is easier with low-air-loss than with air-fluidized beds. Except in settings with special contract rental fees, air-fluidized beds are more expensive than low-air-loss beds. For these reasons, clinicians generally prefer low-air-loss beds for individuals who need a specialized support surface. A randomized controlled trial will be required to compare low-air-loss bed and air-fluidized bed therapy.

When excess moisture on intact skin is a potential source of maceration and skin breakdown, a support surface that provides airflow can be important in drying the skin and preventing additional pressure ulcers. (Strength of Evidence = C.)

Moist skin is more likely to abrade and blister (Leyden, 1984; Leyden, Katz, Stewart, et al., 1977; Zimmerer, Lawson, and Calvert, 1986). When using support surfaces that increase airflow across the patient's skin (e.g., air-fluidized beds and low-air-loss beds), the caregiver should follow manufacturers' instructions for using linens and underpads. When patients are lying on this type of support surface, they should not wear adult incontinence briefs, because these briefs obstruct airflow to the skin.

While Sitting

Positioning techniques and support surfaces for patients who are sitting are important factors in the management of tissue loads.

Positioning Techniques

A patient who has a pressure ulcer on a sitting surface should avoid sitting. If pressure on the ulcer can be relieved, limited sitting may be allowed. (Strength of Evidence = C.)

Interface pressure between the ischial tuberosities and seating surfaces is high and must be relieved frequently to prevent soft tissue damage (Drummond, Narechania, Rosenthal, et al., 1982). Individuals whose sensation is impaired cannot perceive ischemic pain and thus lack a natural defense against pressure ulcers. Those whose mobility is impaired are unable to reposition themselves independently. Thus, both groups depend on outside resources to either relieve pressure for them or remind them to relieve pressure (Merbitz, King, Bleiberg, et al., 1985). As a result, they are prone to numerous episodes of prolonged, unrelieved pressure and should avoid sitting unless pressure over the pressure ulcer can be totally relieved.

Consider postural alignment, distribution of weight, balance, stability, and pressure relief when positioning sitting individuals. (Strength of Evidence = C.)

So that individuals with pressure ulcers can participate in activities of daily living, leisure activities, and personal interactions, a seat must provide more than pressure relief. If the seating surface interferes with these pursuits, individuals are less likely to use the device and thus lack the protection necessary for maintaining healthy skin. Seating considerations to promote maximum personal autonomy and a healthy lifestyle include proper postural alignment and distribution of weight, balance and stability, and pressure relief (Hobson, 1992; Park, 1992). Proper postural alignment reduces the risk for deformities that could compromise respiratory function as well as self-care activities. Proper distribution of weight over the seating surface influences the person's ability to transfer from the seat, defines the magnitude and location of maximum pressure, and allows the load to be transferred to areas that can better tolerate the mechanical loading (Bush, 1969; Drummond, Breed, and Narechania, 1985). Balance and stability directly influence mobility, energy expenditure, and function performance.

Reposition the sitting individual so the points under pressure are shifted at least every hour. If this schedule cannot be kept or is inconsistent with overall treatment goals, return the patient to bed. Individuals who are able should be taught to shift their weight every 15 minutes. (Strength of Evidence = C.)

Research on the etiology of pressure ulcers has indicated that prolonged, uninterrupted mechanical loading of the tissue leads to its breakdown (Kosiak, 1959; Reddy and Cochran, 1979). According to the pressure–time curve developed by Brand (1976), the interface pressure produced during sitting should be relieved at least every hour and preferably at shorter intervals. Clinical practitioners who work with spinal cord–injured patients report that weight shifts are often effective for preventing pressure ulcer formation (Krouskop, Noble, Garber, et al., 1983).

Support Surfaces

Select a cushion based on the specific needs of the individual who requires pressure reduction in a sitting position. Avoid donut-type devices. (Strength of Evidence = C.)

On the basis of the results of animal experiments (Lindan, 1961; Reddy and Cochran, 1979), reducing mechanical loading on the tissue through the use of pressure-reducing devices can diminish the risk for pressure ulcer formation (DeLateur, Berni, Hangladarom, et al., 1976; Ferguson-Pell, Cochran, Cardi, et al., 1986; Garber, Krouskop, and Carter, 1978). For optimal effectiveness, the device must be individually prescribed based on the individual's contour and anatomy and must not interfere with other aspects of mobility and personal autonomy. Pressure-reducing devices allow the individual increased latitude when pressure relief must be provided (for example, when pushups must be done) and in the timing of nursing care schedules.

Ring cushions (donuts) are known to cause venous congestion and edema, although few studies have been carried out to document their deleterious effects. In a study of at-risk patients, Crewe (1987) found that ring cushions are more likely to cause pressure ulcers than to prevent them.

Develop a written plan for the use of positioning devices. (Strength of Evidence = C.)

This recommendation is consistent with usual clinical practice. The use of positioning devices for wheelchair users has been endorsed by several authors (Hamilton, Quek, Lew, et al., 1989; King and French, 1990).

4 Ulcer Care

Initial care of the pressure ulcer involves debridement, wound cleansing, the application of dressings, and possibly adjunctive therapy. In some cases, operative repair will be required (see Chapter 6). In all cases, specific wound care strategies should be consistent with overall patient goals.

Figure 4 depicts the procedural flow, decision points, and preferred management path for ulcer care. The four basic components of an effective ulcer care plan are (1) debridement of necrotic tissue as needed on initial and subsequent assessments (Node 1); (2) cleansing the wound initially and with each dressing change (Node 2); (3) prevention, diagnosis, and treatment of infection (Node 3) (see recommendations in Chapter 5, Managing Bacterial Colonization and Infection, and see Figure 5); and (4) using a dressing that keeps the ulcer bed continuously moist and the surrounding intact tissue dry (Node 4).

Ulcer healing should be assessed at least weekly and the efficacy of the basic ulcer care plan evaluated (Node 5). If the ulcer is healing, it should be monitored (Skip to Node 13). If the ulcer is not healing, the treatment plan should be reassessed and the level of adherence to the plan evaluated. The plan and implementation strategy should be modified as necessary (Node 6).

Electrical stimulation therapy may be considered for patients with Stage III or IV pressure ulcers that are refractory to more conventional treatments. To date, this therapy has been limited to a small number of research centers. Clinicians considering electrical stimulation therapy should ensure that they have proper equipment and trained personnel who are following protocols shown to be effective and safe in appropriately designed and properly conducted clinical trials.

If the ulcer is still not healing (Node 7), selected patients may be candidates for operative repair (Node 8). Information regarding available operative procedures and the anticipated benefits and harms of each procedure should be part of patient counseling and decisionmaking (Node 9). If surgery is preferred, the operative repair procedure most appropriate for the individual should be used (Node 10). Vigilant postoperative followup care is essential to successful operative repair (Node 11). (See Chapter 6, Operative Repair of Pressure Ulcers, for specific recommendations.)

All pressure ulcers that are managed medically should be evaluated at least weekly. All patients with an operative repair should be evaluated at least daily (Node 12). Healing ulcers and surgical wounds should be monitored regularly to ensure continued progress toward the goal of complete healing (Node 13). The frequency of monitoring should be determined by the clinician based on the condition of the patient, the condition of the ulcer, the rate of healing, and the type of health care setting. If progress in healing cannot be demonstrated, the treatment plan must be reassessed and the level

Figure 4. Ulcer care

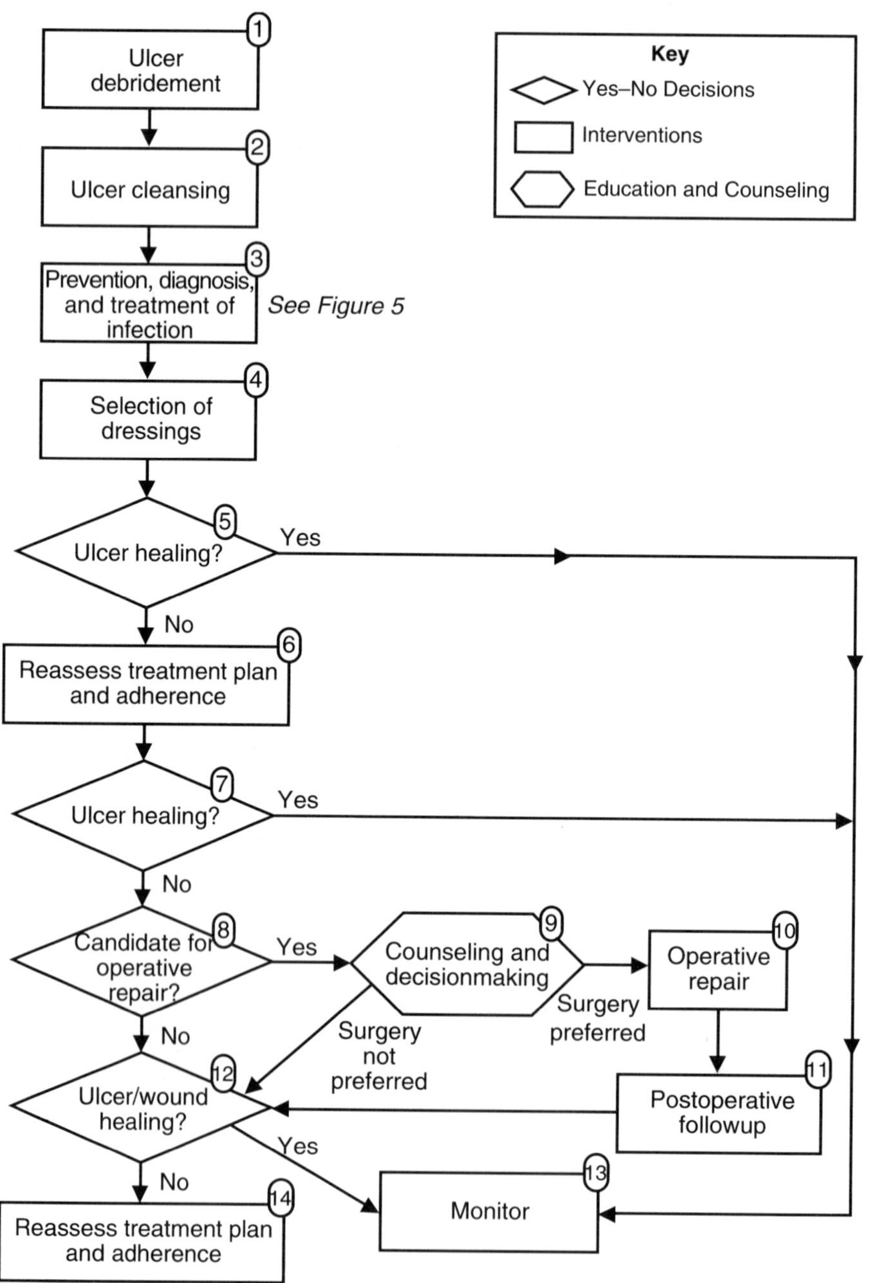

of adherence to that plan evaluated. The plan and implementation strategy should be modified as necessary (Node 14).

Debridement

Moist, devitalized tissue supports the growth of pathological organisms. Therefore, the removal of such tissue favorably alters the healing environment of a wound. Although debridement is a time-honored modality for treating pressure ulcers, it has not been studied in a randomized trial.

Remove devitalized tissue in pressure ulcers when appropriate for the patient's condition and consistent with patient goals. (Strength of Evidence = C.)

Removal of devitalized tissue is considered necessary for wound healing (Agren and Stromberg, 1985; Black and Black, 1987; Boxer, Gottesman, Bernstein, et al., 1969). Moist, necrotic tissue provides a medium for infection (Galpin, Chow, Bayer, et al., 1976; Reuler and Cooney, 1981), initiates an inflammatory response (Longe, 1986; Mummery and Richardson, 1979), places a phagocytic demand on the wound, and retards wound healing. Because these devitalized tissues are avascular, systemic antibiotics are of limited value.

Select the method of debridement most appropriate to the patient's condition and goals. Sharp, mechanical, enzymatic, and/or autolytic debridement techniques may be used when there is no urgent clinical need for drainage or removal of devitalized tissue. If there is urgent need for debridement, as with advancing cellulitis or sepsis, sharp debridement should be used. (Strength of Evidence = C.)

Sharp debridement involves the use of a scalpel, scissor, or other sharp instrument to remove devitalized tissue. The use and benefits of sharp debridement are based on expert opinion (Bale and Harding, 1990; Barrett and Klibanski, 1973; Longe, 1986; Michocki and Lamy, 1976). Sharp debridement should be used to remove areas of thick, adherent eschar and devitalized tissue in extensive ulcers. As the most rapid form of debridement, sharp debridement is urgently indicated when there are signs of advancing cellulitis or sepsis.

Those performing sharp debridement should have demonstrated the necessary clinical skills and should meet licensing requirements. Small wounds can be debrided at the bedside, whereas extensive wounds are usually debrided in the operating room or in a special procedures room. Extensive Stage IV wounds often require debridement in the operating room. When such is required, the surgeon should consider a bone biopsy during the same procedure to determine whether osteomyelitis is present. The need to control pain should be considered.

Mechanical debridement includes the use of wet-to-dry dressings at prescribed intervals, hydrotherapy, wound irrigation, and dextranomers.

All these methods can be used as the initial form of debridement, while the patient is being prepared for surgery, or as the sole form of debridement. Because no studies have addressed the benefits, risks, or efficacy of any of the forms of mechanical debridement, these recommendations are based on expert opinion.

Wet-to-dry dressings adhere to devitalized tissue. Once the dressings are dry—usually within 4 to 6 hours—they can be removed and the devitalized tissue will be removed along with them. The debriding function of the dressing is at least partly defeated if the dressing is moistened prior to removal. One disadvantage of wet-to-dry dressings is that they are nonselective; they remove both nonviable and viable tissues and are therefore potentially traumatic to granulation tissue and especially to new epithelial tissue (Alvarez, Mertz, and Eaglstein, 1983; Longe, 1986; Torrance, 1983). Adequate analgesia should be provided when this method is used (Black and Black, 1987). Once the wound is clean and granulating, moist dressings can be used to promote healing by secondary intention (see recommendations on dressings in this chapter) or the wound can be repaired surgically (see Chapter 6, Operative Repair of Pressure Ulcers).

Hydrotherapy and wound irrigation can be used to debride wounds and soften eschar (Salyer, 1988). Wound irrigation with a safe and effective device such as a 35-mL syringe with a 19-gauge angiocatheter attached to it will provide enough force to remove eschar, bacteria, and other debris (Stevenson, Thacker, Rodeheaver, et al., 1976). A bulb syringe may produce too little pressure for this purpose, whereas some irrigation devices produce too much pressure, damaging healthy tissue. See the cleansing section of this chapter for irrigation pressures delivered by various devices.

Dextranomers are beads that are placed into a wound bed to absorb exudate, bacteria, and other debris. One disadvantage of their use is that they may be difficult to apply if the patient cannot be positioned so that they can be poured into the wound. In addition, the beads are expensive. Furthermore, if dextranomer beads spill onto the floor, a slick surface is created that may be hazardous to both patients and caregivers. In one study of the use of dextranomers, healing time did not appear to decrease greatly (from 25 to 21 days) (Shand and McClemont, 1979).

Enzymatic debridement is accomplished by applying topical debriding agents to devitalized tissues on the wound surface. This option should be considered when individuals cannot tolerate surgery or are in long-term care facilities or receiving care at home, and when the ulcer does not appear to be infected. If infection spreads beyond the ulcer (e.g., advancing cellulitis, sepsis), there is urgent need for sharp debridement. Collagenase, an FDA-licensed biologic, is an example of such a product. Research findings indicate that collagenase promotes debridement and growth of granulation tissue within 3 to 30 days (Boxer, Gottesman, Bernstein, et al., 1969; Lee and Ambrus, 1975; Rao, Sane, and Georgiev, 1975; Varma, Bugatch, and German, 1973). Enzymes can be used alone to break down the eschar, after sharp debridement, or in conjunction with mechanical debridement. Health care providers should refer to specific product information regarding their use.

Autolytic debridement involves the use of synthetic dressings to cover a wound and allow devitalized tissue to self-digest from enzymes normally present in wound fluids. Research supporting the use of autolytic debridement is limited to one animal study (Lydon, Hutchinson, Rippon, et al., 1989) and a small, uncontrolled clinical trial (Carr and Lalagos, 1990). Although autolytic debridement takes longer than other methods, expert clinical opinion indicates that it is an appropriate choice for patients who cannot tolerate other forms of debridement and who are not likely to become infected if their wound is not debrided by other, more rapid means. Autolytic debridement is contraindicated if the ulcer is infected.

Use clean, dry dressings for 8 to 24 hours after sharp debridement associated with bleeding; then reinstitute moist dressings. Clean dressings may be used in conjunction with mechanical or enzymatic debridement techniques. (Strength of Evidence = C.)

The use of dry dressings for the first 8 to 24 hours after sharp debridement tends to limit bleeding. Thereafter, a moist environment should be recreated to support healing. For a rationale supporting the use of clean (as opposed to sterile) dressings, see Chapter 5, Managing Bacterial Colonization and Infection.

Heel ulcers with dry eschar need not be debrided if they do not have edema, erythema, fluctuance, or drainage. Assess these wounds daily to monitor for pressure ulcer complications that would require debridement (e.g., edema, erythema, fluctuance, drainage). (Strength of Evidence = C.)

Stable heel ulcers with a protective eschar covering are considered an exception to the recommendation that all eschar be debrided. Literature is not available on this subject; however, it is the panel's opinion that a wound is stable if it is clean, dry, nontender, nonfluctuant, nonerythematous, and nonsuppurative. The eschar provides a natural protective cover. If any signs of complications appear, however, debridement is usually mandatory.

Prevent or manage pain associated with debridement as needed. (Strength of Evidence = C.)

Although formal studies on this subject are lacking, clinicians report anecdotally that patients complain of pain during debridement. Until such research can be carried out, clinicians should institute measures to prevent, assess, and manage debridement-associated pain. Readers are referred to *Acute Pain Management: Operative or Medical Procedures and Trauma. Clinical Practice Guideline, No. 1,* and to Chapter 2 of this document for specific approaches to this problem.

Wound Cleansing

Wound healing is optimized and the potential for infection is decreased when all necrotic tissue, exudate, and metabolic wastes are removed from the wound. The process of cleansing a wound involves selecting both a wound-cleansing solution and a mechanical means of delivering that solution to the wound. The benefits of obtaining a clean wound must be weighed against the potential trauma to the wound bed as a result of such cleansing. Routine wound cleansing should be accomplished with a minimum of chemical and mechanical trauma.

Cleanse wounds initially and at each dressing change. (Strength of Evidence = C.)

Optimal healing cannot proceed until all inflammatory foreign material is removed from the wound. Materials on the wound surface such as foreign bodies, residual topical agents, dressing residue, wound exudate, and metabolic wastes can be removed by careful wound cleansing (Jones and Shires, 1974; Westaby, 1987).

Use minimal mechanical force when cleansing the ulcer with gauze, cloth, or sponges. (Strength of Evidence = C.)

Traumatized wounds are more susceptible to infection and are slower to heal. Coarse wound-cleansing materials elicit more friction trauma and wound infection than do less coarse ones (Rodeheaver, Smith, Thacker, et al., 1975).

Do not clean ulcer wounds with skin cleansers or antiseptic agents (e.g., povidone iodine, iodophor, sodium hypochlorite solution [Dakin's® solution], hydrogen peroxide, acetic acid). (Strength of Evidence = B.)

Antiseptic agents are reactive chemicals that are cytotoxic to normal tissue. Betadine®, Hibiclens®, pHisoHex®, benzalkonium chloride, and Granulex® have been found to be toxic to human fibroblasts (Custer, Edlich, Prusak, et al., 1971; Johnson, White, and McAnalley, 1989; Rodeheaver, Kurtz, Kircher, et al., 1980; Rydberg and Zederfeldt, 1968).

Skin cleansers contain chemicals that are cytotoxic to wound tissue and should not be used as wound cleansers. Studies have shown that most wound cleansers need to be diluted to maintain cell viability (Burkey, Weinberg, and Brenden, 1993; Foresman, Payne, Becker, et al., 1993). Foresman, Payne, Becker, et al. (1993) studied the required amounts of dilution needed for various skin and wound cleansers to maintain white blood cell viability and phagocytic function. They found a wide range of toxicities among available skin and wound-cleansing agents (see Table 2).

Use normal saline for cleansing most pressure ulcers. (Strength of Evidence = C.)

Table 2. Toxicity index for wound and skin cleansers

Test Agent	Toxicity Index[a]
Shur Clens®	1:10
Biolex™	1:100
Saf Clens™	1:100
Cara Klenz™	1:100
Ultra Klenz™	1:1,000
Clinical Care™	1:1,000
Uni Wash®	1:1,000
Ivory Soap® (0.5 percent)	1:1,000
Constant Clens™	1:10,000
Dermal Wound Cleanser	1:10,000
Puri-Clens™	1:10,000
Hibiclens®	1:10,000
Betadine® Surgical Scrub	1:10,000
Techni-Care™ Scrub	1:100,000
Bard™ Skin Cleanser	1:100,000
Hollister™	1:100,000

[a] The dilution required to maintain white blood cell viability and phagocytic efficiency.
Source: Foresman, Payne, Becker, et al., 1993.

Normal saline is the preferred cleansing agent because it is physiologic, will not harm tissue, and adequately cleanses most wounds. Wounds with adherent materials may benefit from the use of those commercial wound cleansers that do not contain harmful chemicals. Available wound cleansers range widely from safe to toxic. Commercial wound cleansers contain surfactants and other chemicals intended to enhance their efficacy, and some of these chemicals may have deleterious effects on wound cells (Bryant, Rodeheaver, Reem, et al., 1984; Foresman, Payne, Becker, et al., 1993). Commercial wound cleansers do not require FDA approval for distribution.

Use enough irrigation pressure to enhance wound cleansing without causing trauma to the wound bed. Safe and effective ulcer irrigation pressures range from 4 to 15 psi. Table 3 indicates the irrigation pressure delivered by various clinically available devices. (Strength of Evidence = B.)

If irrigation pressures are too low (below 4 psi), they will not cleanse the wound adequately. Several investigators found that pressurized irrigation more effectively removed wound bacteria and debris than did gravity or bulb syringe irrigation (Brown, Shelton, Bornside, et al., 1978; Green, Carlson, Briggs, et al., 1971; Gross, Cutright, and Bhaskar, 1972; Hamer, Robson, Krizek, et al., 1975). An irrigation pressure of 8 psi effectively cleanses the wound and reduces the risk of trauma and wound infection. A 35-mL syringe with a 19-gauge needle or angiocatheter delivers saline to the wound at 8 psi and was found to be significantly more effective in removing bacteria and preventing infection than was a bulb syringe (Stevenson, Thacker, Rodeheaver, et al., 1976). Irrigation at 13 psi was significantly superior to a bulb syringe in reducing wound inflammation in

Table 3. Irrigation pressures delivered by various devices

Device	Irrigation Impact Pressure (psi)
Spray Bottle—Ultra Klenz™ [a] (Carrington Laboratories, Inc., Dallas TX)	1.2
Bulb Syringe [a] (Davol Inc., Cranston, RI)	2.0
Piston Irrigation Syringe (60-mL) with catheter tip (Premium Plastics, Inc., Chicago, IL)	4.2
Saline Squeeze Bottle (250-mL) with irrigation cap (Baxter Healthcare Corp., Deerfield, IL)	4.5
Water Pik® at lowest setting (#1) (Teledyne Water Pik, Fort Collins, CO)	6.0
Irrijet® DS Syringe with tip (Ackrad Laboratories, Inc., Cranford, NJ)	7.6
35-mL syringe with 19-gauge needle or angiocatheter	8.0
Water Pik® at middle setting (#3) [b] (Teledyne Water Pik, Fort Collins, CO)	42
Water Pik® at highest setting (#5) [b] (Teledyne Water Pik, Fort Collins, CO)	>50
Pressurized Cannister-Dey-Wash™ [b] (Dey Laboratories, Inc., Napa, CA)	>50

[a] These devices may not deliver enough pressure to adequately cleanse wounds.
[b] These devices may cause trauma and drive bacteria into wounds. They are not recommended for cleansing of soft-tissue wounds.
Source: Beltran, Thacker, and Rodeheaver, 1994.

traumatic wounds (Longmire, Broom, and Burch, 1987). Wound irrigation pressures of 10 and 15 psi were superior to those of 1 or 5 psi (Rodeheaver, Pettry, Thacker, et al., 1975). Irrigation pressures that exceed 15 psi may cause trauma to the wound and drive bacteria into the tissue (Bhaskar, Cutright, and Gross, 1969; Wheeler, Rodeheaver, Thacker, et al., 1976). Such high pressures lead to fluid dispersion and extensive penetration of irrigation fluid into the wound tissue.

Consider whirlpool treatment for cleansing pressure ulcers that contain thick exudate, slough, or necrotic tissue. Discontinue whirlpool when the ulcer is clean. (Strength of Evidence = C.)

Increasing the length of time a wound surface is in contact with water during whirlpool therapy may enhance the removal of debris from the pressure ulcer. Feedar and Kloth (1990) recommend twice-daily whirlpool cleansing to remove debris and residue. Neiderhuber, Stribley, and Koepke (1975) and Bohannon (1982) found in separate studies that whirlpool treatment followed by a clean pressurized rinse was more effective in removing bacteria than was whirlpool alone. Wound trauma can occur, however, if the wound is positioned too close to the high-pressure water jets in the whirlpool. Whirlpool treatment should be discontinued when the ulcer is considered clean, because the benefits of wound cleansing are outweighed by the potential for trauma to the regenerating tissue as a result of the agitating water (Feedar and Kloth, 1990).

Dressings

Pressure ulcers require dressings to maintain their physiologic integrity. An ideal dressing should protect the wound, be biocompatible, and provide ideal hydration. The condition of the ulcer bed and the desired dressing function determine the type of dressing needed. The cardinal rule is to keep the ulcer tissue moist and the surrounding intact skin dry.

Use a dressing that will keep the ulcer bed continuously moist. Wet-to-dry dressings should be used only for debridement and are not considered continuously moist saline dressings. (Strength of Evidence = B.)

Several investigators studied pressure ulcer healing outcomes by comparing dry wound healing techniques with moist ones. Kurzuk-Howard, Simpson, and Palmieri (1985) compared heat lamp treatments with film dressings, and Saydak (1990) compared dry gauze dressings with absorptive powder treatment. Several investigators compared wet-to-dry gauze dressings with various moist wound-healing alternatives (Fowler and Goupil, 1984; Gorse and Messner, 1987; Sebern, 1986). The results of these studies suggest that the rate of healing is better with the moist wound-healing treatment than with dressings or treatments that dry the wound bed.

Use clinical judgment to select a type of moist wound dressing suitable for the ulcer. Studies of different types of moist wound dressings showed no differences in pressure ulcer healing outcomes. (Strength of Evidence = B.)

In five controlled trials in which moist saline gauze and other types of moist wound dressings were compared, no significant differences were noted in pressure ulcer healing outcomes (Alm, Hornmark, Fall, et al., 1989; Colwell, Foreman, and Trotter, 1992; Neill, Conforti, Kedas, et al., 1989; Oleske, Smith, White, et al., 1986; Xakellis and Chrischilles, 1992). On the basis of these results, clinicians may select a suitable dressing that supports moist wound healing.

Choose a dressing that keeps the surrounding intact (periulcer) skin dry while keeping the ulcer bed moist. (Strength of Evidence = C.)

Moisture makes intact skin more susceptible to injury. Various techniques can be used to protect the skin from drainage resulting from incontinence and other sources of excessive moisture (Panel for the

Prediction and Prevention of Pressure Ulcers in Adults, 1992). Patients with pressure ulcers have additional sources of moisture (wound drainage and wound treatment solutions) that may damage unprotected skin.

Choose a dressing that controls exudate but does not desiccate the ulcer bed. (Strength of Evidence = C.)

Exudative ulcers were found to heal more slowly than nonexudative ones (Gorse and Messner, 1987; Xakellis and Chrischilles, 1992). Although wounds heal better in a moist environment, excessive exudate can macerate surrounding tissue. According to expert opinion, excessive exudate should be absorbed away from the ulcer bed. Several case series report that some dressings work very well for highly exudative wounds. When absorptive dressings are used to remove excess exudate, care should be taken not to desiccate the ulcer bed.

Consider caregiver time when selecting a dressing. (Strength of Evidence = B.)

In five studies that compared the nursing time required to care for pressure ulcer patients treated with moist saline gauze dressings and patients treated with film or hydrocolloid dressings, the former approach took significantly more time than the latter (Alm, Hornmark, Fall, et al., 1989; Colwell, Foreman, and Trotter, 1992; Neill, Conforti, Kedas, et al., 1989; Sebern, 1986; Xakellis and Chrischilles, 1992). This difference relates to the fact that film or hydrocolloid dressings need to be changed less often. However, time spent in assessing whether the dressing remains intact between changes of film or hydrocolloid dressings was not studied. Whether the time taken to assess the dressing results in differences in the overall cost in the hospital or nursing home setting depends on the cost of the dressing materials versus the cost of nursing time. In the home setting, caregivers may choose more expensive dressing materials to reduce the frequency of dressing changes.

Eliminate wound dead space by loosely filling all cavities with dressing material. Avoid overpacking the wound. (Strength of Evidence = C.)

Wound cavities need to be filled so that areas do not "wall off" and become abscessed. Overpacking a wound may increase pressure on the tissue in the wound bed, potentially causing additional tissue damage (Maklebust and Sieggreen, 1991).

Monitor dressings applied near the anus, since they are difficult to keep intact. (Strength of Evidence = C.)

A number of investigators reported that both film and hydrocolloid dressings failed to remain intact near the anus, and thus their effectiveness was difficult to evaluate (Ahmed, 1982; Dobrzanski, Kelly, Gray, et al.

1990; Goren, 1989; Lingner, Rolstad, Wetherill, et al., 1984). Dobrzanski, Kelly, Gray, et al. (1990) also reported that hydrocolloid dressings over the sacral area tended to roll when the subject changed position. Clinicians report that "picture-framing" or taping the edges of the dressing may reduce this problem.

Adjunctive Therapies

The roles of several adjunctive therapies in enhancing pressure ulcer healing have been investigated. The therapies considered by the panel included electrical stimulation; hyperbaric oxygen; infrared, ultraviolet, and low-energy laser irradiation; ultrasound; miscellaneous topical agents (including cytokine growth factors); and systemic drugs other than antibiotics. At this time, electrical stimulation is the only adjunctive therapy with sufficient supporting evidence to warrant recommendation by the panel.

Consider a course of treatment with electrotherapy for Stage III and IV pressure ulcers that have proved unresponsive to conventional therapy. Electrical stimulation may also be useful for recalcitrant Stage II ulcers. (Strength of Evidence = B.)

Data from five clinical trials, involving a total of 147 patients, support the effectiveness of electrotherapy in enhancing the healing rate of pressure ulcers that have been unresponsive to conventional therapy (Carley and Wainapel, 1985; Feedar, Kloth, and Gentzkow, 1991; Gentzkow, Pollack, Kloth, et al., 1991; Griffin, Tooms, Mendius, et al., 1991; Kloth and Feedar, 1988). This finding was consistent across a variety of electrical stimulation protocols. Adverse reactions were limited to minor uncomfortable tingling sensations in 15 percent of patients in one study. Most of the subjects enrolled in these studies had Stage III or IV ulcers.

To date, this therapy has been limited to a small number of research centers. Clinicians considering electrical stimulation therapy should ensure that they have proper equipment and trained personnel who are following protocols shown to be effective and safe in appropriately designed and properly conducted clinical trials.

The therapeutic efficacy of hyperbaric oxygen; infrared, ultraviolet, and low-energy laser irradiation; and ultrasound has not been sufficiently established to permit recommendation of these therapies for the treatment of pressure ulcers. (Strength of Evidence = C.)

Studies of the efficacy of hyperbaric oxygen in pressure ulcer healing have been limited to case series employing topical hyperbaric oxygen (Fisher, 1969; Rosenthal and Schurman, 1971). The lack of controlled clinical trials, combined with in vitro evidence suggesting topical hyperbaric oxygen does not increase tissue oxygen tension beyond the superficial dermis (Gruber, Heitkamp, Billy, et al., 1970), precludes the panel from making any recommendation for the treatment of pressure ulcers. The use of various forms of light (infrared, ultraviolet, and low-energy laser) to promote wound healing has been reported in the literature (Freytes, Fernandez, and Fleming, 1965; Kahn, 1984; MacKinnon and Cleek, 1984; Mester, Mester, and Mester, 1985; Scott, 1983; Stillwell, 1971; Surinchak, Alago, Bellamy, et al., 1983; Wills, Anderson, Beattie, et al., 1983). Controlled clinical trials are generally lacking, however, and data specific to pressure ulcers are minimal. The efficacy of ultrasound for healing of pressure ulcers was evaluated in one controlled trial (McDiarmid, Burns, Lewith, et al., 1985), which showed an improved rate of healing for infected ulcers, but no difference for clean ulcers. The marginal benefit demonstrated in this study and the lack of additional controlled trials of pressure ulcers prevented formulation of any recommendation.

The therapeutic efficacy of miscellaneous topical agents (e.g., sugar, vitamins, elements, hormones, other agents), growth factors, and skin equivalents has not yet been sufficiently established to warrant recommendation of these agents at this time. (Strength of Evidence = C.)

Agents reviewed for this section included some that are very old and some that are new. Of the older agents, sugar, honey, zinc, magnesium, gold, aluminum, phenytoin, aloe vera gel, yeast extract, and insulin all have been popular for short periods of time. Some of these agents are currently being used and investigated. Zinc acetate and aluminum hydroxide ointment (Motta, 1991) and phenytoin (El Zayat, 1989) were evaluated in a controlled and blinded fashion. Many of the newer agents such as cytokine growth factors (e.g., recombinant platelet-derived growth factor-BB [rPDGF-BB] and basic fibroblast growth factor [bFGF]) and skin equivalents are currently being scrutinized in clinical trials. The use of rPDGF-BB (Robson, Phillips, Thomason, et al., 1992a, 1992b) and bFGF (Robson, Phillips, Lawrence, et al., 1992) has been evaluated in a controlled and blinded fashion. All the studies listed above have shown encouraging results, but data that adequately address the efficacy of any of these agents in the treatment of pressure ulcers are limited. Therefore, for now, none of these agents can be recommended for this purpose. However, it should not be construed that these agents do not deserve further study or that an agent's efficacy might not be demonstrated in trials now under way.

The therapeutic efficacy of systemic agents other than antibiotics has not been sufficiently established to permit their recommendation for the treatment of pressure ulcers. (Strength of Evidence = C.)

The panel considered several nonantibiotic systemic drugs (i.e., vasodilators, hemorrheologics [pentoxiphylline], serotonin inhibitors, fibrolytic agents) as potential adjunctive therapies for pressure ulcer treatment. Preliminary reports suggest that systemic vasodilators may improve skin ulcer outcomes associated with scleroderma (Baron, Skrinskas, Urowitz, et al., 1982) and peripheral vascular disease (Olsson, 1980). A case series indicates that pentoxiphylline may be of benefit in the treatment of diabetic ulcers (Adler, 1991). No data, however, support the use of systemic vasodilators, hemorrheologics, serotonin inhibitors, or fibrolytic agents in treating pressure ulcers.

5 Managing Bacterial Colonization and Infection

Stage II, III, and IV pressure ulcers are invariably colonized with bacteria. In most cases, adequate cleansing and debridement prevent bacterial colonization from proceeding to the point of clinical infection. Recommendations regarding the management of colonization and infection are provided below. Figure 5 guides the clinician through a preferred pathway for managing ulcer colonization and local and systemic infection.

Pressure Ulcer Colonization and Infection

Minimize pressure ulcer colonization and enhance wound healing by effective wound cleansing and debridement. (Strength of Evidence = A.) If purulence or foul odor is present, more frequent cleansing and possibly debridement are required. (Strength of Evidence = C.)

Several quantitative bacteriological studies found a direct correlation between high levels of bacteria in pressure ulcers and failure to heal (Bendy, Nuccio, Wolfe, et al., 1964; Daltrey, Rhodes, and Chattwood, 1981; Lyman, Tenery, and Basson, 1970; Sapico, Ginunas, Thornhill-Joynes, et al., 1986). High levels of bacteria are found in wounds that contain necrotic tissue (Sapico, Ginunas, Thornhill-Joynes, et al., 1986). Foul odor in a pressure ulcer is usually associated with the presence of anaerobic organisms (Sapico, Ginunas, Thornhill-Joynes, et al., 1986). Effective wound cleansing and debridement remove the debris that supports bacterial growth and delays wound healing.

Do not use swab cultures to diagnose wound infection, because all pressure ulcers are colonized. (Strength of Evidence = C.)

All open pressure ulcers are colonized with bacteria. Routine swab cultures detect only the surface contaminants and may not truly reflect the organism(s) causing the tissue infection (Rousseau, 1989). The level of bacteria in the ulcer tissue must be determined in order to document the presence of wound infection (Krizek and Robson, 1975). As recommended by the CDC, this can be accomplished by culture of fluid obtained by needle aspiration or biopsy of ulcer tissue (Garner, Jarvis, Emori, et al., 1988).

Consider initiating a 2-week trial of topical antibiotics for clean pressure ulcers that are not healing or are continuing to produce exudate after 2 to 4 weeks of optimal patient care (as defined in this guideline). The antibiotic should be effective against gram-negative, gram-positive, and anaerobic organisms (e.g., silver sulfadiazine, triple antibiotic). (Strength of Evidence = A.)

Figure 5. Managing bacterial colonization and infection

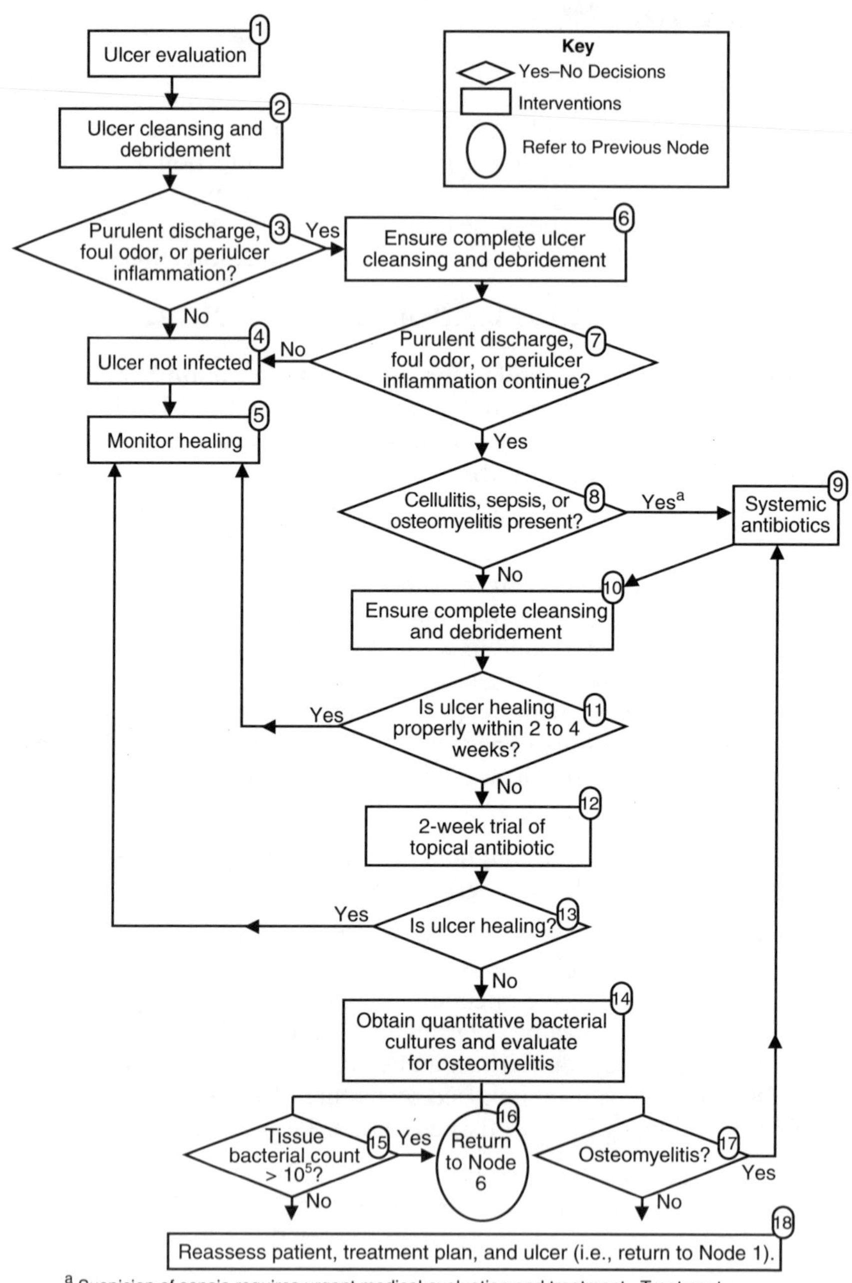

[a] Suspicion of sepsis requires urgent medical evaluation and treatment. Treatment of sepsis is not discussed in this guideline.

Data from two clinical trials support the effectiveness of topical antibiotics in reducing the levels of bacteria in pressure ulcers to 10^5 organisms per gram of tissue or less (Bendy, Nuccio, Wolfe, et al., 1964; Kucan, Robson, Heggers, et al., 1981). This decrease in bacterial count was accompanied by decisive improvement in the clinical appearance of the wound, consistent with progression toward healing. Case study reports of allergic sensitization and other adverse reactions suggest the need for close monitoring during this treatment (Johnson, 1988; Schechter, Wilkinson, and Del Carpio, 1984).

Perform quantitative bacterial cultures of the soft tissue and evaluate the patient for osteomyelitis when the ulcer does not respond to topical antibiotic therapy. (Strength of Evidence = C.)

Several studies documented that when the bacterial content in an ulcer exceeds 10^5 organisms per gram of tissue, healing is impaired (Bendy, Nuccio, Wolfe, et al., 1964; Daltrey, Rhodes, and Chattwood, 1981; Lyman, Tenery, and Basson, 1970; Sapico, Ginunas, Thornhill-Joynes, et al., 1986). The level of bacteria in the ulcer tissue can best be determined by tissue biopsy (Garner, Jarvis, Emori, et al., 1988; Robson, 1991). The CDC recommends culture by tissue biopsy or fluid obtained by needle aspiration (Garner, Jarvis, Emori, et al., 1988).

Other studies suggested that approximately 25 percent of nonhealing pressure ulcers have underlying osteomyelitis (Allman, 1989; Lewis, Bailey, Pulawski, et al., 1988; Sugarman, 1984). Although numerous methods have been used to evaluate the bone underlying a pressure ulcer, the "gold standard" for diagnosing osteomyelitis is pathological examination of a bone biopsy specimen (Lewis, Bailey, Pulawski, et al., 1988; Sugarman, 1987). However, most experts have been reluctant to perform an immediate bone biopsy unless an extensive operative debridement procedure is to be performed anyway. Numerous strategies for noninvasive diagnosis of osteomyelitis have been reported. Lewis, Bailey, Pulawski, et al. (1988) reported that bone scans are rarely useful in practice because of their high false-positive rate. They suggested using instead a combination of three tests (white blood cell count, erythrocyte sedimentation rate, and plain x-ray); if all three tests were positive, the positive predictive value for osteomyelitis was 69 percent. The positive and negative predictive values of CT scan or magnetic resonance imaging (MRI) in diagnosing osteomyelitis under pressure ulcers were not reported in the literature.

Do not use topical antiseptics (e.g., povidone iodine, iodophor, sodium hypochlorite [Dakin's® solution], hydrogen peroxide, acetic acid) to reduce bacteria in wound tissue. (Strength of Evidence = B.)

No controlled studies have documented that repeated topical application of antiseptics to the surface of chronic wounds significantly decreases the level of bacteria within the wound tissue. Numerous studies, however, have documented the toxic effects of exposing wound-healing cells to antiseptics (Fleming, 1919; Lineaweaver, Howard, Soucy, et al., 1985; Teepe, Koebrugge, Lowik, et al., 1993).

Institute appropriate systemic antibiotic therapy for patients with bacteremia, sepsis, advancing cellulitis, or osteomyelitis. (Strength of Evidence = A.) Systemic antibiotics are not required for pressure ulcers with only clinical signs of local infection. (Strength of Evidence = C.)

Bacteremia, sepsis, advancing cellulitis, and osteomyelitis are systemic infections that cannot be successfully treated with further cleansing or debridement and require systemic antibiotics. The details of treatment for these conditions are not discussed in this guideline; however, a brief overview is provided below.

Bacteremia and sepsis associated with pressure ulcers are commonly caused by *Staphylococcus aureus*, gram-negative rods, or *Bacteroides fragilis*. If patients with pressure ulcers develop clinical signs of sepsis (e.g., unexplained fever, tachycardia, hypotension, deterioration in mental status), urgent medical attention is required. It is appropriate to rule out other causes of the symptoms, obtain blood cultures, and treat with antibiotics that will cover these organisms (Bryan, Dew, and Reynolds, 1983; Chow, Galpin, and Guze, 1977; Galpin, Chow, Bayer, et al., 1976; Lewis, Bailey, Pulawski, et al., 1988). According to one study, mortality is higher if patients are not treated with appropriate antibiotics (Chow, Galpin, and Guze, 1977). As a consequence, patients with clinical signs of ulcer-related sepsis must be treated with antibiotics that will cover the organisms noted above. Obtaining blood cultures will allow the initial empirical treatment regimen to be focused and simplified if the causative organism(s) can be identified.

Advancing cellulitis is indicative of invasive tissue infection. It should be treated with appropriate antibiotics.

Osteomyelitis is an infectious complication of pressure ulcers that can result in delayed healing, more extensive tissue damage, a longer length of hospitalization, and higher mortality rates (Allman, 1989; Lewis, Bailey, Pulawski, et al., 1988; Sugarman, 1984). Early recognition and effective treatment of osteomyelitis are critical. Invasive and noninvasive diagnostic strategies have been discussed. Although cleansing and debridement are important aspects of treatment, long-term systemic antibiotic therapy is essential (Aust and Page, 1985; Longe, 1986; Pearlman, McShane, Jochimsen, et al., 1976).

Protect pressure ulcers from exogenous sources of contamination (e.g., feces). (Strength of Evidence = C.)

One study confirmed that fecal incontinence is associated with slower rates of pressure ulcer healing (Ferrell, Osterweil, and Christenson, 1993). Exposure to feces increases the level of bacterial colonization in a pressure ulcer.

Infection Control

Follow body substance isolation (BSI) precautions or an equivalent system appropriate for the health care setting and the patient's condition when treating pressure ulcers. (Strength of Evidence = C.)

BSI is a system of infection-control procedures routinely used with all patients to prevent cross-contamination of pathogens. The system emphasizes the use of barrier precautions to isolate potentially infectious body substances (Lynch, Cummings, Roberts, et al., 1990). According to Lynch, Jackson, Cummings, et al. (1987), BSI has six components:

1. Wear gloves for anticipated contact with blood, secretions, mucous membranes, nonintact skin, and moist body substances for all patients. Change gloves before treating another patient. Handwashing between patients is essential.
2. After other types of patient contact, wash the hands for 10 seconds with soap and friction to remove transient microbial flora, and then rinse with running water (Garner and Favero, 1986).
3. Wear additional barriers such as gowns, plastic aprons, masks, or goggles when moist body substances (secretions, blood, or body fluids) are likely to soil the clothing or the skin or splash in the face. The panel notes that protective eyewear, mask (or a faceshield that covers the eyes and face), gloves, and in some cases protective gowns should be used for pressure ulcer irrigation when there is reasonable expectation that wound secretions might be aerosolized.
4. Place soiled reusable articles and linen, as well as trash, in containers that are securely sealed to prevent leaking. Double bagging is not necessary unless the outside of the bag is visibly soiled.
5. Place needles (without recapping them) and sharp instruments in puncture-resistant, rigid containers. If such containers are not available, recapping using the one-hand technique is acceptable.
6. Assign to private rooms those patients with diseases that could be transmitted by the airborne route (e.g., pulmonary tuberculosis) and other diseases listed under precautions for strict isolation in the category-specific isolation (Center for Disease Control, 1970). The use of private rooms is also indicated for those patients likely to soil articles in their environment with body substances.

In addition, the panel recognizes the potential for transmitting infection through whirlpool equipment. Whirlpool equipment should be disinfected between patients. For guidance regarding effective disinfection techniques, clinicians may consult the Association for Practitioners in Infection Control

(APIC) guideline regarding the selection and use of disinfectants (Rutala, 1990).

Use clean gloves for each patient. When treating multiple ulcers on the same patient, attend to the most contaminated ulcer last (e.g., in the perianal region). Remove gloves and wash hands between patients. (Strength of Evidence = C.)

One set of gloves can be used on the same patient with multiple pressure ulcers. Hands must be washed and gloves changed between patients. No research evidence at this time supports the need to change gloves when caring for multiple ulcers on the same patient.

Use sterile instruments to debride pressure ulcers. (Strength of Evidence = C.)

To avoid introducing additional bacteria into an open wound when tissue integrity is disrupted during debridement, sterile instruments, as opposed to clean ones, should be used in hospitals, long-term care facilities, and nursing homes. Followup after debridement should include monitoring the patient's temperature and being alert for signs of bacteremia or sepsis (e.g., unexplained fever, tachycardia, hypotension, deterioration in mental status).

Use clean dressings, rather than sterile ones, to treat pressure ulcers, as long as dressing procedures comply with institutional infection-control guidelines. (Strength of Evidence = C.)

The fear of cross-contamination of microorganisms within institutions is realistic. Therefore, each institution should establish and rigorously adhere to procedures to prevent cross-contamination. There is no evidence to indicate that the use of sterile dressings results in a better outcome.

Infection-control procedures should include strict adherence to BSI and good handwashing between patients. Multipatient treatment carts that are taken to the bedside should not be used to house dressing supplies. Individual patients should have their own dressing supplies that are protected from inadvertent environmental contamination by water damage, dust accumulation, or contact contaminants. "Clean," bundled dressings can be purchased less expensively than can individual dressings; however, measures should be taken to ensure that they remain clean. Such measures include keeping dressings in the original package or in other plastic packaging; storing them in a clean, dry place; and discarding the entire package if any of the dressings become wet, contaminated, or dirty. Dressings, instruments, and solutions should be obtained from suppliers who can ensure that shipment and handling will not expose the dressings and supplies to water damage, pest and rodent contamination, or gross soiling. Caregivers must wash their hands before contact with the supply of clean dressings or dressing supplies. Prior to the dressing or treatment, only the number of dressings necessary for each dressing change should be removed from containers. Once the hands of the caregiver are soiled with wound secretions, they should not come in contact with the remaining clean dressings and other supplies until the gloves are removed and hands are washed.

Clean dressings may also be used in the home setting. Disposal of contaminated dressings in the home should be done in a manner consistent with local regulations. (Strength of Evidence = C.)

Clean dressings, as opposed to sterile ones, are recommended for home use until research demonstrates otherwise. This recommendation is in keeping with principles regarding nosocomial infections and with past success of clean urinary catheterization in the home setting and takes into account the expense of sterile dressings and the dexterity required to apply them. The "no-touch" technique can be used for dressing changes. This technique is a method of changing surface dressings without touching the wound or the surface of any dressing that might be in contact with the wound. Adherent dressings should be grasped by the corner and removed slowly, whereas gauze dressings can be pinched in the center and lifted off.

The Environmental Protection Agency recommends that soiled dressings be placed in securely fastened plastic bags before being added to other household trash (Environmental Protection Agency, 1993; Simmons, Trusler, Roccaforte, et al., 1990). Local regulations vary, however, and home care agencies and patients are advised to follow procedures that are consistent with local laws.

6 Operative Repair of Pressure Ulcers

Operative procedures to repair pressure ulcers include one or more of the following: Direct closure, skin grafting, skin flaps, musculocutaneous flaps, and free flaps. Although more research is needed to develop clear criteria for selecting those individuals most likely to benefit from surgical management, the panel has provided some general criteria. Preoperative patient counseling should include information about the operative procedures available and the anticipated benefits and potential risks of each. Factors that might impair healing should be addressed preoperatively. Vigilant postoperative followup is considered essential to healing and prevention of recurrence.

Patient Selection

Determine patient need and suitability for operative repair when clean Stage III or Stage IV pressure ulcers do not respond to optimal patient care (as defined in this guideline). Possible candidates are medically stable and adequately nourished and can tolerate operative blood loss and postoperative immobility. Quality of life, patient preferences, treatment goals, risk of recurrence, and expected rehabilitative outcome are additional considerations. (Strength of Evidence = C.)

Surgical repair can be used to provide a skin covering or to establish durable soft-tissue coverage. Flaps containing muscle are effective in managing osteomyelitis because they provide a physiologic barrier to infection, eliminate dead space in the wound, and improve vascularity. Increased vascularity increases local oxygen tension, enhances the delivery of systemic antibiotics, and improves lymphocyte function (Anthony, Huntsman, and Mathes, 1992; Becker, 1979; Bruck, Buttemeyer, Grabosch, et al., 1991).

Operative procedures may last 1 to 3 hours and may result in a blood loss of up to 1,500 mL. Therefore, patients with medical conditions that would be worsened by anesthesia, blood loss, systemic stress, or immobility following surgery are usually not candidates for repair. Adequate nutrition is essential for wound healing. Several laboratory parameters can be used to assist in evaluating the patient's nutritional status, including serum levels of hemoglobin, transferrin, and albumin and lymphocyte counts. See Chapter 2, Assessment, for a complete discussion of nutritional assessment.

Surgical repair of Stage IV ulcers is common because flaps provide more durable tissue than does scar tissue. One decision analysis suggests that surgery would be favored for repair of Stage III ulcers in nursing home residents with moderate dementia unless the rate of operative success was below 30 percent or the projected rate of healing with conservative management was over 40 percent. Although operative repair was $17,000 more costly than conservative treatment, it would improve 1-year survival rates in this population (Siegler and Lavizzo-Mourey, 1991). This cost analysis assumes continued residence at the nursing home. Average healing time was reported to decrease from 12.8 weeks with skin grafts to 4.8 weeks with musculocutaneous flaps (Anthony, Huntsman, and Mathes, 1992).

In contrast, the rate of healing for medically managed Stage III ulcers in nursing home patients was 14 percent at 6 weeks (Berlowitz and Wilking, 1990), 31.5 percent at 3 months, and 58.9 percent at 6 months (Brandeis, Morris, Nash, et al., 1990). Conservative medical management resulted in healed wounds in 23.3 percent of Stage IV pressure ulcers at 3 months and in 33.2 percent at 6 months (Brandeis, Morris, Nash, et al., 1990).

Controlling Factors That Impair Healing

Promote successful surgical closure by controlling or correcting factors that may be associated with impaired healing, such as smoking, spasticity, levels of bacterial colonization, incontinence, and urinary tract infection. (Strength of Evidence = C.)

The carbon monoxide and nicotinic acid found in cigarette smoke act as potent vasoconstrictors, compromising arterial inflow to flaps used for operative repair. Smoking also aggravates ischemia by increasing blood viscosity (Read, 1984). In addition, the neutrophils in smokers release excessive amounts of oxidase, which damages tissues and small vessels (Fincham, 1992). The longer the patient can stop smoking before surgery the better; however, it may be 6 weeks before improvements in immune response can be noted (Jones, 1985–86). Cessation for 12 to 24 hours prior to surgery will reduce carbon monoxide and nicotinic acid levels. Nicotine patches should not be used, since their half-life is twice that of smoked tobacco (Fincham, 1992). Although patients would not be denied operative repair just because they choose to continue smoking or cannot stop smoking, they should be counseled about the risk of flap failure (Lewis, 1989).

Spasticity and mass reflex in paraplegic patients may facilitate transfer, but severe spasticity hinders healing after surgery (Herceg and Harding, 1978). Ulcer cleansing may increase spasticity because it acts as a noxious stimulus triggering a spastic reflex (Hall and Young, 1983). After surgery, spasticity can put tension on wound edges and lead to dehiscence. Joint or muscle contracture may require surgical release to decrease wound tension (Haher, Haher, Devlin, et al., 1983).

Levels of bacterial colonization in the wound can be controlled and urinary incontinence can be managed with urinary catheters to decrease the risk of wound infection. Urinary tract infection is a common cause of sepsis. Although many clinicians administer perioperative antibiotics prophylactically (Salzberg, Gray, Petro, et al., 1990), there are no research data to support the efficacy of this practice. See Chapter 5, Managing Bacterial Colonization and Infection, and Chapter 4, Ulcer Care.

Operative Procedures

Use the most effective and least traumatic method to repair the ulcer defect. Wounds can be closed by direct closure, skin grafting, skin flaps, musculocutaneous flaps, and free flaps. To minimize recurrence, the choice of operative technique is based on the individual patient's needs and overall goals. (Strength of Evidence = C.)

Repair of Stage III and IV ulcers requires tissue that will provide bulk, be resistant to pressure, and withstand normal wear and tear. In planning the reconstruction, the clinician begins by determining the simplest technique that will best restore missing tissue and blood supply without sacrificing function. Operative procedures are listed below in order of increasing complexity. Refer to Operative Repair in the Glossary for additional information.

- **Direct closure.** Although the simplest method of pressure ulcer repair would be direct closure with sutures, this approach stretches the skin and creates tension that frequently leads to dehiscence, especially when the patient moves (Lewis, 1989). Thus, primary closure with a suture is seldom used except for small, superficial ulcers (Anthony, Huntsman, and Mathes, 1992).
- **Skin grafts.** Skin grafts are the next simplest method of wound closure and are used to repair shallow pressure ulcers. Skin grafts, however, provide only a skin barrier. When applied to granulating bone, skin grafts quickly erode, precluding healing (Nuseibeh, 1974; Sundell, Pentti, and Langenskiold, 1967).
- **Skin flaps.** Prior to the 1970's, repair using local skin flaps was the standard surgical treatment for ulcers. Today, they are not usually employed for primary repair but are used instead as alternatives for secondary repair (Sanchez, Eamegdool, and Conway, 1969). Local skin flaps have a random vascular supply, and the tissue used for repair is often a redistribution of inadequately perfused tissue rather than a planned revascularization using specific blood vessels. Although some random flaps have a good blood supply, that supply may not be in the zone of injury.
- **Musculocutaneous flaps.** Musculocutaneous flaps are usually the best choice for paraplegic patients or when loss of muscle function does not contribute to comorbidity. For ambulatory patients the choice is less clear, since the improved blood supply and reliability of the muscle flap must be balanced against the need to sacrifice functional muscle units (Koshima, Moriguchi, Soeda, et al., 1993; Kroll and Rosenfield, 1988; Vyas, Binns, and Wilson, 1980). Musculocutaneous flaps can help heal osteomyelitis and limit the damage caused by shearing, friction, and pressure (Daniel, Hall, and MacLeod, 1979; Mathes, Feng, and Hunt, 1983; Vasconez, Schneider, and Jurkiewicz, 1977).

- **Free flaps.** Free flaps are muscle-type flaps in which the vein and artery are disconnected at the donor site and reconnected to the vessels at the recipient site with the aid of a microscope. This is the most complex method of wound closure, and it has not been described in the literature for closure of pressure ulcers.

One recent finding in the literature is on the use of tissue expansion techniques, by which surrounding tissues are stretched and rotated to cover pressure ulcers. Advantages of this adjunctive method appear to be that local tissue can be used for operative repair, the three-dimensional expander temporarily provides equal distribution of pressure, and the tissue can be expanded on an outpatient basis. Long-term results are not yet known (Braddom and Leadbetter, 1989; Esposito, Di Caprio, Ziccardi, et al., 1991; Gray, Salzberg, Petro, et al., 1990; Yuan, 1989).

Before recommending a specific operative technique, the clinician will also consider the site of the ulcer. Site-specific considerations are discussed for sacral, ischial, trochanteric, and more extensive pressure ulcers.

- **Sacral ulcers.** The gluteus maximus is a large muscle that can be used in its entirety or in portions to repair pressure ulcers over the sacrum. Since its vascular supply is ample, use of one portion of the gluteus maximus does not devascularize other portions of the muscle. Disadvantages to its use are that it may be difficult to identify in quadriplegic patients due to atrophy, flap dissection may be bloody, and the flaps are bulky. The gluteus maximus serves as the primary extender, external rotator, and abductor of the hip; therefore, the whole muscle cannot be used as a flap in ambulatory patients without sacrificing hip function (Fisher, Arnold, Waldorf, et al., 1983; Ger and Levine, 1976; Heywood and Quaba, 1989; Minami, Mills, and Pardoe, 1977; Parkash and Banerjee, 1986; Parry and Mathes, 1982; Scheflan, Nahai, and Boswick, 1981). Several types of secondary flaps can be used for operative repair of sacral ulcers (Bailey, 1971; Hill, Brown, and Jurkiewicz, 1978; Lewis, 1989).

- **Ischial ulcers.** Ischial ulcers can be repaired by using the inferior gluteus maximus musculocutaneous flap. A disadvantage of this approach is that flap advancement requires lateral division of the gluteus maximus muscle, which is contraindicated in an ambulatory patient. Short-term complications were related to flap viability, and ulcer recurrence was uncommon at the site of repair (Baek, Williams, McElhinney, et al., 1980; Lewis, 1989; Maruyama, Ohnishi, and Takeuchi, 1984; Parkash and Banerjee, 1986; Scheflan, Nahai, and Boswick, 1981). The tensor fascia lata (TFL) can also be used for repair (Abramsohn, Murphy, Pandeya, et al., 1981; Lewis, Cunningham, and Hugo, 1981; McGregor and Buchan, 1980). In patients with a sensory loss below L3-4, the TFL flap can be used to provide sensation. Favorable outcomes reported were sensation in the perianal region and improved bowel control (Cochran, Edstrom, and Dibbell, 1981; Coleman and Jurkiewicz, 1984; Daniel, Terzis, and Cunningham, 1976; Krupp, Kuhn, and Zaech, 1983; Luscher, de Roche, Krupp, et al., 1991; Spear, Kroll, and Little, 1987).

- **Trochanteric ulcers.** Trochanteric ulcers are difficult to repair surgically for several reasons. Incisions needed for local skin flaps may interfere with the design of future flaps to repair other ulcers. In contrast to most other common pressure ulcer sites, the bony prominence beneath a trochanteric ulcer is mobile rather than stationary, which tends to create large areas of undermining and make the adherence of a skin flap difficult. The TFL flap is the first choice of musculocutaneous flaps to repair trochanteric ulcers. Advantages to using the TFL are that the muscle is near the ulcer site, has a consistent vascular pedicle, can provide sensation, is moved easily, and is an expendable muscle. One disadvantage is that a dog-ear deformity is often created (Daniel and Faibisoff, 1982; Daniel, Hall, and MacLeod, 1979; McGregor and Buchan, 1980; Micali and Romeo, 1982; Muguti, 1990; Paletta, Freedman, and Shehadi, 1989; Siddiqui, Wiedrich, and Lewis, 1993). Other musculocutaneous flaps used for repair include the vastus lateralis muscle flap with skin graft coverage (Bovet, Nassif, Guimberteau, et al., 1982; Minami, Hentz, and Vistnes, 1977), the inferior-based gluteus (Becker, 1979; Parkash and Banerjee, 1986), the sartorius (Maruyama and Hamano, 1978), the rectus femoris (Peters, Cartotto, Morris, et al., 1991), and the vastus lateralis (Tolhurst, 1980).

- **Extensive pressure ulcers.** Extensive pressure ulcers are defined as those that cannot heal on their own and cannot be closed with a single musculocutaneous flap. Several procedures have been discussed in the literature, including a thigh flap (Lawton and De Pinto, 1987; Royer, Pickrell, Georgiade, et al., 1969; Rubayi, Pompan, and Garland, 1991; Sagi, Meller, Kon, et al., 1987; Yanai, Bandoh, and Tsuzuki, 1991); skin flaps from the lower leg, with preservation of the upper leg (Burkhardt, 1972; Chen, Weng, and Noordhoff, 1986; Holman, 1985); and translumbar amputation (hemicorporectomy) (Aust and Page, 1985; Pearlman, McShane, Jochimsen, et al., 1976; Terz, Schaffner, Goodkin, et al., 1990).

Prophylactic ischiectomy is not recommended because it often results in perineal ulcers and urethral fistulas, which are more threatening problems than ischial ulcers. (Strength of Evidence = C.)

Although ischiectomy had been advocated for the treatment as well as the prevention of ischial ulcers (Arregui, Canon, Murray, et al., 1965), recent studies report perineal ulcer occurrence and the development of urethral fistula after this procedure (Hackler and Zampieri, 1987; Karaca, Binns, and Blumenthal, 1978). The ulcers are caused by pressure diverted to the remaining ischium or anterior pelvis.

Postoperative Care

Minimize pressure to the operative site by use of an air-fluidized bed, a low-air-loss bed, or a Stryker frame for a minimum of 2 weeks. Assess postoperative viability of the surgical site as clinically indicated. Have the patient slowly increase periods of time sitting or lying on the flap to increase its tolerance to pressure. To determine the degree of tolerance, monitor the flap for pallor, redness, or both that do not resolve after 10 minutes of pressure relief. Ongoing patient education is imperative to reduce the risk of recurrence. (Strength of Evidence = C.)

No studies have focused solely on postoperative care and rehabilitation after pressure ulcer repair; therefore, the information in this section is based on expert opinion. Complications of flap reconstruction have included hematoma, wound separation, flap necrosis, flap dehiscence, infection, and seroma (Vasconez, Schneider, and Jurkiewicz, 1977). To reduce the risk of hematoma and seroma, wound suction devices are left in the wound for about 1 week or until drainage is minimal. Many complications are due to insufficient blood supply to the flap. Use of pressure-relieving beds allows the patient to lie on the flap without interfering with tissue perfusion. The head of an air-fluidized bed should not be elevated above 15 degrees from the horizontal. Although some clinicians prefer to place patients in a prone position, complications of this position include airway difficulties (especially in quadriplegic patients), ulnar nerve compression (Nath and Taylor, 1978), confusion, and boredom. When the patient's position is changed, the flap should not be subjected to friction or shear.

Following sacral ulcer repair, fecal contamination of the wound should be avoided. This can be accomplished by using constipating medications and a low-fiber diet (Black and Black, 1987; Rubayi, Cousins, and Valentine, 1990).

Rehabilitation of the patient with a flap includes progressively longer periods of sitting, with flap viability checked after each sitting period. Flap viability may be compromised if pallor, redness, or both at the operative site do not decrease after 10 minutes of pressure relief (Bih and Lu, 1989). Patients are taught to shift their body weight once they are bearing weight on the flap and to inspect the skin daily using a mirror. See Chapter 3, Managing Tissue Loads, for more specific recommendations on techniques for positioning and pressure reduction when the patient is sitting or in bed.

Assess for recurrence of pressure ulcers as an ongoing component of care. Caregivers should provide education and encourage adherence to measures for pressure reduction, daily skin examination, and intermittent relief techniques. (Strength of Evidence = A.)

Recurrence rates for pressure ulcers following operative repair range from 13 percent (Mandrekas and Mastorakos, 1992) to 56 percent (Relander and Palmer, 1988). Carelessness and noncompliance are important risk factors for recurrence (Disa, Carlton, and Goldberg, 1992; Morgan, 1976).

Disa, Carlton, and Goldberg (1992) compared ulcer recurrence after surgery in various groups of patients. The incidence of new ulcers in the traumatic, paraplegic group was 79 percent, compared with 29 percent in the nontraumatic, nonparaplegic group (which consisted mainly of elderly nursing home residents), and 0 percent in the nontraumatic paraplegic group. Adequate social support was associated with lack of recurrence, and substance abuse was related to recurrence.

Recurrence rates may be reduced with the use of sensate flaps. More important, however, is the development of programs in ulcer prevention, with emphasis on patient education and adherence. The long-term preventive value of musculocutaneous flap coverage of pressure ulcers must be continually reevaluated in a large series of patients.

7 Education and Quality Improvement

Institutions and agencies concerned with health care are responsible for developing and implementing educational programs designed to translate knowledge about pressure ulcers into effective treatment strategies. The goals of such programs are to promote the healing and prevent the deterioration of existing pressure ulcers and to prevent new ones.

The goal of quality improvement is to develop and implement a systematic, interdisciplinary, and ongoing quality improvement (QI) program for facilitating comprehensive, consistent care that can be monitored, evaluated, and changed as patient conditions and current knowledge warrant.

Education

Recommendations for developing and implementing educational programs are provided in the following categories: Prevention and treatment, assessing tissue damage, and monitoring outcomes.

Prevention and Treatment: A Continuum

Design, develop, and implement educational programs for patients, caregivers, and health care providers that reflect a continuum of care. The program should begin with a structured, comprehensive, and organized approach to prevention and should culminate in effective treatment protocols that promote healing as well as prevent recurrence. (Strength of Evidence = C.)

Education is the means by which current knowledge about pressure ulcers can be translated into effective strategies for prevention and treatment. Clinicians and scientists alike often include the words "prevention" and "treatment" (or "management") in the titles of their published works, indicating that they see these two concepts as inextricably linked (Byrne and Feld, 1984; Droessler and Maibusch, 1979; Gould, 1986). Although only one study has demonstrated that education (of caregivers) alone was responsible for reducing the incidence or severity of pressure ulcers in a group of hospitalized patients (Moody, Fanale, Thompson, et al., 1988), many investigators have incorporated structured educational programs into a total pressure ulcer management program, with skin integrity the desirable outcome of both preventive and treatment efforts (Distel, 1981; Sachs and Mathews, 1990). Some educational programs include extensive protocols for both prevention and treatment of pressure ulcers (Law, 1990), and others advocate practicing or teaching prevention during the treatment phase (Hamilton, Quek, Lew, et al., 1989). Even though developing and implementing programs that address both prevention and treatment of pressure ulcers may prove time-consuming, this two-pronged approach is essential to maintaining skin integrity and preventing recurrent ulcers.

Develop educational programs that target appropriate health care providers, patients, family members, and caregivers. Present information at an appropriate level for the target audience to maximize retention and ensure a carryover into practice. Use principles of adult learning (e.g., explanation, demonstration, questioning, group discussion, drills). (Strength of Evidence = C.)

Information that is presented at an appropriate level for the target audience is more likely to be retained and carried over into practice (Maklebust and Magnan, 1992). Principles of adult learning should be considered when designing educational programs. Specifically, the program should address the learner's needs, interests, background (vocational, educational, cultural), and current knowledge of the material to be presented (Bergevin, Morris, and Smith, 1963; Verduin, Miller, and Greer, 1977). Objectives should be clear because they provide direction for the learner and teacher as well as content for program development. A clear set of objectives will also allow the instruction and learning to be evaluated. Techniques that work especially well with the adult learner include (but are not limited to) explanation, demonstration, questioning, group discussion, drills, and inquiry (Warren, 1977).

Involve the patient and caregiver, when possible, in pressure ulcer treatment and prevention strategies and options. Include information on pain, discomfort, possible outcomes, and duration of treatment, if known. Encourage the patient to actively participate in and comply with decisions regarding pressure ulcer prevention and treatment. (Strength of Evidence = C.)

Studies have shown that compliance is greater and treatment more successful when the patient participates actively in the process of learning (Andberg, Rudolph, and Anderson, 1983; Barnes, 1987; Engstrand, 1979; LaMantia, Hirschwald, Goodman, et al., 1987). It is recommended that, whenever possible, the patient understand the variety, availability, and relevance of treatment options and participate in decisions regarding management of the pressure ulcer. Information on pain, discomfort, possible outcomes, and, if known, duration of treatment should be included (Morison, 1989; Rottkamp, 1976; Sebern, 1987).

Educational programs should identify those responsible for pressure ulcer treatment and describe each person's role. The information presented and the degree of participation expected should be appropriate to the audience. (Strength of Evidence = C.)

These programs should include specific, accurate, and reliable information about pressure ulcer treatment as well as about appropriate educational methods. Nurses are the target audience in most of the works cited in the literature on the subject (Bates-Jensen, 1990; Dealey, 1991; Distel, 1981; Gosnell and Pontius, 1988; Gould, 1985; Green and Katz, 1991; Miller and Rantz, 1989; Sachs and Mathews, 1990, Van Ness, 1989). Health care providers from other disciplines would also benefit from such educational programs. The levels of caregiver training, education, and experience in any one facility will vary. The protocols for pressure ulcer treatment must be developed with consideration for the specific group or level of caregiver who will be assigned to carry out the protocols.

Assessing Tissue Damage

Educational programs should emphasize the need for accurate, consistent, and uniform assessment, description, and documentation of the extent of tissue damage. (Strength of Evidence = C.)

The most frequently cited content area in teaching protocols and educational programs that address the treatment of pressure ulcers is accurate and consistent assessment, description, and documentation of the extent to which tissue is damaged. Accurate staging and description of the pressure ulcer are a prerequisite to development and implementation of appropriate, effective treatment protocols and to effective, ongoing monitoring of tissue healing (Bolton and van Rijswijk, 1991; Hamilton, Quek, Lew, et al., 1989; Phipps, Bauman, Berner, et al., 1984; Sebern, 1987). To provide effective treatment, caregivers must understand clearly the extent of the tissue damage (Brewer, 1989; French and Ledwell-Sifner, 1991; Sachs and Mathews, 1990). Accurate staging of the ulcer is a prerequisite to development and implementation of appropriate, effective treatment protocols.

Include the following information when developing an educational program on the treatment of pressure ulcers (Strength of Evidence = C):

- **Etiology and pathology.**
- **Risk factors.**
- **Uniform terminology for stages of tissue damage based on specific classification.**
- **Principles of wound healing.**
- **Principles of nutritional support with regard to tissue integrity.**
- **Individualized program of skin care.**
- **Principles of cleansing and infection control.**
- **Principles of postoperative care including positioning and support surfaces.**
- **Principles of prevention to reduce recurrence.**

- **Product selection (i.e., categories and uses of support surfaces, dressings, topical antibiotics, or other agents).**
- **Effects or influence of the physical and mechanical environment on the pressure ulcer, and strategies for management.**
- **Mechanisms for accurate documentation and monitoring of pertinent data, including treatment interventions and healing progress.**

The first step in planning treatment is accurate assessment of the wound. As can be seen from the foregoing list, other essential components of an effective educational program include risk factors and risk assessment; uniform terminology and documentation; individualized skin care; principles of wound cleansing and infection control; and categories and uses of dressings, medications, and support surfaces (Andberg, Rudolph, and Anderson, 1983; Arikian, Kingery, Beall, et al., 1990; Barnes, 1987; Bolton and van Rijswijk, 1991; Braden and Bryant, 1990; Droessler and Maibusch, 1979; Irvine and Black, 1990; Iverson-Carpenter, 1988).

Update educational programs on an ongoing and regular basis to integrate new knowledge, techniques, or technologies. (Strength of Evidence = C.)

Educational programs should be ongoing, presented regularly, and updated frequently. New technologies for the treatment of pressure ulcers are being developed constantly, with many new products now being marketed for cleansing, dressing, and debriding these lesions as well as for providing pressure relief. In many cases these products have not undergone rigorous testing, and, therefore, their effectiveness remains unconfirmed. In addition, many clinicians are uninformed or misinformed about the implications of research designed to identify and analyze proposed treatment strategies (Gould, 1985, 1986). A continuing educational effort is essential to ensure that current information is presented and that knowledge has been retained.

Monitoring Outcomes

Evaluate the effectiveness of an educational program in terms of measurable outcomes: Implementation of guideline recommendations, healing of existing ulcers, reducing the incidence of new or recurrent ulcers, and preventing the deterioration of existing ulcers. (Strength of Evidence = C.)

Evaluation of outcomes should serve as the basis for changing existing practice and improving care. The effectiveness of educational programs designed to teach assessment and treatment techniques must also be evaluated (Andberg, Rudolph, and Anderson, 1983). Therefore, mechanisms for testing both the knowledge gained and the skills mastered should be an integral part of the educational program (Anderson and Andberg, 1980). Periodic followup will enhance the audience's ability to retain information and improve their skills (Arikian, Kingery, Beall, et al., 1990). Improvements in outcomes depend on knowledgeable nurses and other health care providers who will provide care according to a specific, individualized, and documented plan.

Include a structured, comprehensive, and organized educational program as an integral part of quality improvement monitoring. Use information from quality assurance/improvement surveys to identify deficiencies, to evaluate the effectiveness of care, and to determine the need for education and policy changes. Focus inservice training on identified deficiencies. (Strength of Evidence = C.)

QI surveys can be used to obtain information about the effectiveness of nursing care and the need for additional education or policy changes (Van Ness, 1989). If deficiencies are identified, inservice training can focus on those specific areas (Droessler and Maibusch, 1979). Knowledgeable nurses and ongoing updated inservice education and training are essential if measurable improvements are to be achieved (Gosnell and Pontius, 1988; Miller and Rantz, 1989; VanEtten, Sexton, and Smith, 1990). The results of quality improvement monitoring should serve as the basis for changing practice protocols and improving care.

Quality Improvement

Recommendations follow on QI to facilitate comprehensive, consistent care of pressure ulcers.

Obtain intradepartmental and interdepartmental QI support for pressure ulcer management as a major aspect of care. (Strength of Evidence = C.)

Support within and between departments is essential for a coordinated and comprehensive program. Support must be provided by clinical departments as well as nonclinical ones such as data management, utilization management, medical records, purchasing, pharmacy, and central supply in order to generate and utilize useful information (Baranoski, 1992).

Convene an interdisciplinary committee of interested and knowledgeable persons to address QI in pressure ulcer management. (Strength of Evidence = C.)

The committee may be convened initially to plan for pressure ulcer prevention rather than treatment. Since pressure ulcer management is a multifactorial, multidisciplinary problem, an interdisciplinary team is essential. Team members may include (but not be limited to) the QI coordinator, clinical nurse specialist, administrator, enterostomal therapy nurse, staff nurses, nutritionist, occupational therapist, physical therapist, geriatrician, and physiatrist. Consultants with special expertise, such as dermatologists or plastic surgeons, may be enlisted as needed. Although team members may vary depending on the type of setting, an interdisciplinary team with consultants can be assembled in acute care settings, long-term care facilities, and home care agencies (Arikian, Kingery, Beall, et al., 1990; Gosnell and Pontius, 1988; LaMantia, Hirschwald, Goodman, et al., 1987).

Identify and monitor the occurrence of pressure ulcers to determine their incidence and prevalence. This information will serve as a baseline to the development, implementation, and evaluation of treatment protocols. (Strength of Evidence = C.)

No data are available to suggest realistic or desirable rates of pressure ulcer prevalence and incidence. Current data vary by setting, such as acute care setting, long-term care facility, and home (via home care agencies); they establish the current status but not what might be achieved with the use of a concerted QI process. On the basis of initial data, goals to maintain the current statistics or improve them should be set by individual institutions and agencies (Arikian, Kingery, Beall, et al., 1990; Bodnar and Myron, 1992; Droessler and Maibusch, 1979).

Monitor the incidence and prevalence of pressure ulcers on a regular basis. (Strength of Evidence = C.)

Baseline data are useful only in initially quantifying the magnitude of the pressure ulcer problem. Regular monitoring is essential in order to track and trend the experience and to evaluate prevention and treatment programs that have been implemented. Several elements should be included in the monitoring process. To the extent possible, data should be collected concurrently rather than retrospectively. Sources of data include direct patient assessment, the medical record, and staff interviews.

Quantitative data elements should include total census, number of patients with pressure ulcers, total number of ulcers, number of ulcers by stage, percentage of ulcers that are nosocomial, and site of ulcers on the body.

Qualitative data may be collected and organized using a structure-process-outcome format. Structure is represented by the availability of supplies, equipment, personnel, and financial support. Process is represented by available standards, policies, procedures, and treatment protocols. Process also includes a documentation system that will facilitate consistent care and the evaluation of that care by means of tracking and trending the patient's skin condition and pressure ulcer characteristics (Blom, 1985; Distel, 1981; Droessler and Maibusch, 1979; Gosnell and Pontius, 1988). Outcomes of care can be measured in terms of the incidence and prevalence of pressure ulcers.

Develop, implement, and evaluate educational programs based on the data obtained from QI monitoring. (Strength of Evidence = C.)

The setting, identification of caregivers, pressure ulcer data, and current information will help guide the content of the educational programs. Although caregiver knowledge of pressure ulcer management is one indicator of the effectiveness of the program, other outcomes should also be emphasized. Thus, caregiver implementation of recommended interventions should be evaluated, as well as measurements of pressure ulcer healing, progression, and prevention (Arikian, Kingery, Beall, et al., 1990; Lubin and Powell, 1991).

References

Abramsohn L, Murphy BJ, Pandeya NK, Stallings JO, Bergman RS. The tensor fascia lata myocutaneous flap: experience with its use as a rotation flap. J Am Osteopath Assoc 1981 Jul;80(11):733–5.

Acute Pain Management Guideline Panel. Acute pain management: operative or medical procedures and trauma. Clinical Practice Guideline, No. 1. Rockville (MD): Agency for Health Care Policy and Research, Public Health Service, US Department of Health and Human Services; 1992 Feb. AHCPR Publication No. 92-0032. 145 p.

Adler PF. Assessing the effects of pentoxifylline (Trental) on diabetic neurotrophic foot ulcers. J Foot Surg 1991 May–Jun;30(3):300–3.

Agren MS, Stromberg HE. Topical treatment of pressure ulcers: a randomized comparative trial of Varidase and zinc oxide. Scand J Plast Reconstr Surg 1985;19(1):97–100.

Ahmed MC. Op-Site for decubitus care. Am J Nurs 1982 Jan;82(1):61–4.

Allman RM. Epidemiology of pressure sores in different populations. Decubitus 1989 May;2(2):30–3.

Allman RM, Laprade CA, Noel LB, Walker JM, Moorer CA, Dear MR, Smith CR. Pressure sores among hospitalized patients. Ann Intern Med 1986 Sep;105(3):337–42.

Allman RM, Walker JM, Hart MK, Laprade CA, Noel LB, Smith CR. Air-fluidized beds or conventional therapy for pressures sores: a randomized trial. Ann Intern Med 1987 Nov;107(5):641–8.

Alm A, Hornmark AM, Fall PA, Linder L, Bergstrand B, Ehrnebo M, Madsen SM, Setterberg G. Care of pressure sores: a controlled study of the use of a hydrocolloid dressing compared with wet saline gauze compresses. Acta Derm Venereol (Stockh) 1989;149 Suppl:1–10.

Alvarez OM, Mertz PM, Eaglstein WH. The effect of occlusive dressings on collagen synthesis and re-epithelialization in superficial wounds. J Surg Res 1983;35(2):142–8.

Ameis A, Chiarcossi A, Jimenez J. Management of pressure sores: comparative study in medical and surgical patients. Postgrad Med 1980 Feb;67(2):177–84.

Andberg MM, Rudolph A, Anderson T. Improving skin care through patient and family training. Top Clin Nurs 1983;5(2):45–54.

Anderson TP, Andberg MM. Psychosocial factors associated with pressure sores. Arch Phys Med Rehabil 1979 Aug;60(8):341–6.

Anderson TP, Andberg MM. An investigation of decubitus ulcer as a manifestation of a psychosocial problem: final report. Minneapolis, (MN): University of Minnesota Health Sciences Center, Department of Medicine and Rehabilitation; 1980. 55 p.

Anthony JP, Huntsman WT, Mathes SJ. Changing trends in the management of pelvic pressure ulcers: a 12-year review. Decubitus 1992 May;5(3):44–7, 50–1.

Arikian VL, Kingery C, Beall K, Abbott R. Education and QA: a model for continuous improvement in skin integrity. J Nurs Qual Assur 1990 Nov;5(1):1–7.

Aronoff GR, Friedman SJ, Doedens DJ, Lavelle KJ. Increased serum iodide concentration from iodine absorption through wounds treated topically with povidone-iodine. Am J Med Sci 1980 May–Jun;279(3):173–6.

Arregui J, Canon B, Murray JE, O'Leary JJ Jr. Long-term evaluation of ischiectomy in the treatment of pressure ulcers. Plast Reconstr Surg 1965 Dec;36(6):583–90.

Aust JB, Page CP. Hemicorporectomy. J Surg Oncol 1985 Dec;30(4):226–30.

Baek SM, Williams GD, McElhinney AJ, Simon BE. The gluteus maximus myocutaneous flap in the management of pressure sores. Ann Plast Surg 1980 Dec;5(6):471–6.

Bailey BN. Surgical closure of sacral sores. Proc R Soc Med 1971 Nov;64(11):1148.

Bale S, Harding KG. Using modern dressings to effect debridement. Prof Nurse 1990;5(5):244–5.

Baranoski S. Collaborative roles lead to success in wound healing. Decubitus 1992 May;5(3):66–8.

Barbenel JC, Jordan MM, Nicol SM, Clark MO. Incidence of pressure-sores in the Greater Glasgow Health Board area. Lancet 1977 Sep 10;2(8037):548–50.

Barnes SH. Patient/family education for the patient with a pressure necrosis. Nurs Clin North Am 1987 Jun;22(2):463–74.

Baron M, Skrinskas G, Urowitz MB, Madras PN. Prostaglandin E1 therapy for digital ulcers in scleroderma. Can Med Assoc J 1982 Jan 1;126(1):42–5.

Barrett D Jr, Klibanski A. Collagenase debridement. Am J Nurs 1973 May;73(5):849–51.

Bates-Jensen B. New pressure ulcer status tool. Decubitus 1990 Aug;3(3):14–5.

Becker H. The distally-based gluteus maximus muscle flap. Plast Reconstr Surg 1979 May;63(5):653–6.

Beltran KA, Thacker JG, Rodeheaver GT. Impact pressures generated by commercial wound irrigation devices. (Unpublished research report). Charlottesville (VA): University of Virginia Health Science Center; 1994.

Bendy RH Jr, Nuccio PA, Wolfe E, Collins B, Tamburro C, Glass W, Martin CM. Relationship of quantitative wound bacterial counts to healing of decubiti: effect of topical gentamicin. Antimicrob Agents Chemother 1964;4:147–55.

Bergevin P, Morris D, Smith RM. Adult education procedures: a handbook of tested patterns for effective participation. New York: Seabury Press; 1963.

Bergstrom N, Braden B. A prospective study of pressure sore risk among institutionalized elderly. J Am Geriatr Soc 1992 Aug;40(8):747–58.

Bergstrom N, Demuth PJ, Braden BJ. A clinical trial of the Braden Scale for Predicting Pressure Sore Risk. Nurs Clin North Am 1987 Jun;22(2):417–28.

Berkwits L, Yarkony GM, Lewis V. Marjolin's ulcer complicating a pressure ulcer: case report and literature review. Arch Phys Med Rehabil 1986 Nov;67(11):831–3.

Berlowitz DR, Wilking SV. Risk factors for pressure sores: a comparison of cross-sectional and cohort-derived data. J Am Geriatr Soc 1989 Nov;37(11):1043–50.

Berlowitz DR, Wilking SV. The short-term outcome of pressure sores. J Am Geriatr Soc 1990 Jul;38(7):748–52.

Bhaskar SN, Cutright DE, Gross A. Effect of water lavage on infected wounds in the rat. J Periodontol 1969 Nov;40(11):671–2.

Bih LI, Lu SY. The rehabilitation of pressure sores after myocutaneous flap surgery. Taiwan I Hsueh Hui Tsa Chih 1989 Apr;88(4):387–93.

Black JM, Black SB. Surgical management of pressure ulcers. Nurs Clin North Am 1987 Jun;22(2):429–38.

Blom MF. Dramatic decrease in decubitus ulcers. Geriatr Nurs (New York) 1985 Mar–Apr;6(2):84–7.

Bodnar B, Myron P. Portrait of practice: reducing the prevalence of pressure ulcers. Decubitus 1992 Mar;5(2):49–52.

Bohannon RW. Whirlpool versus whirlpool rinse for removal of bacteria from a venous stasis ulcer. Phys Ther 1982 Mar;62(3):304–8.

Bolton L, van Rijswijk L. Wound dressings: meeting clinical and biological needs. Dermatol Nurs 1991 Jun;3(3):146–61.

Bovet JL, Nassif TM, Guimberteau JC, Baudet J. The vastus lateralis musculocutaneous flap in the repair of trochanteric pressure sores: technique and indications. Plast Reconstr Surg 1982 May;69(5):830–4.

Boxer AM, Gottesman N, Bernstein H, Mandl I. Debridement of dermal ulcers and decubiti with collagenase. Geriatrics 1969 Jul;24(7):75–86.

Braddom RL, Leadbetter MG. The use of a tissue expander to enlarge a graft for surgical treatment of a pressure ulcer in a quadriplegic: case report. Am J Phys Med Rehabil 1989 Apr;68(2):70–2.

Braden BJ, Bryant R. Innovations to prevent and treat pressure ulcers. Geriatr Nurs 1990 Jul–Aug;11(4):182–6.

Brand PW. Pressure sores—the problem. In: Kenedi RM, Cowden JM, Scales JT, editors. Bed sore biomechanics. London: Macmillan; 1976. p. 19–23.

Brandeis GH, Morris JN, Nash DJ, Lipsitz LA. The epidemiology and natural history of pressure ulcers in elderly nursing home residents. JAMA 1990 Dec 12;264(22):2905–9. [See Comment in: JAMA 1991 Apr 3:265(13):1688.]

Breslow RA, Hallfrisch J, Goldberg AP. Malnutrition in tubefed nursing home patients with pressure sores. J Parenter Enteral Nutr 1991 Nov–Dec;15(6):663–8.

Breslow RA, Hallfrisch J, Guy DG, Crawley B, Goldberg AP. The importance of dietary protein in healing pressure ulcers. J Am Geriatr Soc 1993 Apr;41(4):357–62.

Brewer DJ. Skin care chart development. Ostomy Wound Manage 1989 Spring;22:53–5.

Brown LL, Shelton HT, Bornside GH, Cohn I Jr. Evaluation of wound irrigation by pulsatile jet and conventional methods. Ann Surg 1978 Feb;187(2):170–3.

Bruck JC, Buttemeyer R, Grabosch A, Gruhl L. More arguments in favor of myocutaneous flaps for the treatment of pelvic pressure sores. Ann Plast Surg 1991 Jan;26(1):85–8.

Bryan CS, Dew CE, Reynolds KL. Bacteremia associated with decubitus ulcers. Arch Intern Med 1983 Nov;143(11):2093–5.

Bryant CA, Rodeheaver GT, Reem EM, Nichter LS, Kenney JG, Edlich RF. Search for a nontoxic surgical scrub solution for periorbital lacerations. Ann Emerg Med 1984 May;13(5):317–21.

Burkey JL, Weinberg C, Brenden RA. Differential methodologies for the evaluation of skin and wound cleansers. Wounds 1993;5(6):284–91.

Burkhardt BR. An alternative to the total-thigh flap for coverage of massive decubitus ulcers. Plast Reconstr Surg 1972 Apr;49(4):433–8.

Burr RG. Blood zinc in the spinal patient. J Clin Pathol 1973 Oct;26(10):773–5.

Bush CA. Study of pressures on skin under ischial tuberosities and thighs during sitting. Arch Phys Med Rehabil 1969 Apr;50(4):207–13.

Byrne N, Feld M. Overcoming the red menace: preventing and treating decubitus ulcers. Nursing 1984 Apr;14(4):55–7.

Carley PJ, Wainapel SF. Electrotherapy for acceleration of wound healing: low intensity direct current. Arch Phys Med Rehabil 1985 Jul;66(7):443–6.

Carr RD, Lalagos DE. Clinical evaluation of a polymeric membrane dressing in the treatment of pressure ulcers. Decubitus 1990 Aug;3(3):38–42.

Center for Disease Control (CDC). Isolation techniques for use in hospitals. Atlanta (GA): Center for Disease Control; 1970. Public Health Service Publication No. 2054.

Chen HC, Weng CJ, Noordhoff MS. Coverage of multiple extensive pressure sores with a single filleted lower leg myocutaneous free flap. Plast Reconstr Surg 1986 Sep;78(3):396–8.

Chen LH, Fan-Chiang WL. Biochemical evaluation of riboflavin and vitamin B_6 status of institutionalized and non-institutionalized elderly in central Kentucky. Int J Vitam Nutr Res 1981;51(3):232–8.

Chernoff R, Milton K, Lipschitz D. The effect of a very high-protein liquid formula (Replete®) on decubitus ulcer healing in long-term tube-fed institutionalized patients [abstract]. J Am Diet Assoc 1990;90(9):A–130.

Chow AW, Galpin JE, Guze LB. Clindamycin for treatment of sepsis caused by decubitus ulcers. J Infect Dis 1977 Mar;135 Suppl:S65–8.

Clarke M, Kadhom HM. The nursing prevention of pressure sores in hospital and community patients. J Adv Nurs 1988 May;13(3):365–73.

Cochran JH Jr, Edstrom LE, Dibbell DG. Usefulness of the innervated tensor fascia lata flap in paraplegic patients. Ann Plast Surg 1981 Oct;7(4):286–8.

Coleman JJ 3d, Jurkiewicz MJ. Methods of providing sensation to anesthetic areas. Ann Plast Surg 1984 Feb;12(2):177–86.

Colwell JC, Foreman MD, Trotter JP. A comparison of the efficacy and cost-effectiveness of two methods of managing pressure ulcers. Decubitus 1992 Jul;6(4):28–36.

Conine TA, Choi AK, Lim R. The user-friendliness of protective support surfaces in prevention of pressure sores. Rehabil Nurs 1989 Sep–Oct;14(5):261–3.

Conine TA, Daechsel D, Lau MS. The role of alternating air and Silicore overlays in preventing decubitus ulcers. J Rehabil Res 1990;13(1):57–65.

Crewe RA. Problems of rubber ring nursing cushions and a clinical survey of alternative cushions for ill patients. Care Sci Pract 1987 Jun;5(2):9–11.

Cruz Santiago G, Kaminski MV Jr, Palencia Salinas C. Adequacy of vitamin C supplementation in total parenteral nutrition [abstract]. J Parenter Enteral Nutr 1981;5(6).

Custer J, Edlich RF, Prusak M, Madden J, Panek P, Wangensteen OH. Studies in the management of the contaminated wound: V. An assessment of the effectiveness of pHisoHex and Betadine surgical scrub solutions. Am J Surg 1971 May;121:572–5.

Daltrey DC, Rhodes B, Chattwood JG. Investigation into the microbial flora of healing and non-healing decubitus ulcers. J Clin Pathol 1981 Jul;34(7):701–5.

Daniel RK, Faibisoff B. Muscle coverage of pressure points—the role of myocutaneous flaps. Ann Plast Surg 1982 Jun;8(6):446–52.

Daniel RK, Hall EJ, MacLeod MK. Pressure sores: a reappraisal. Ann Plast Surg 1979 Jul;3(1):53–63.

Daniel RK, Terzis JK, Cunningham DM. Sensory skin flaps for coverage of pressure sores in paraplegic patients: a preliminary report. Plast Reconstr Surg 1976 Sep;58(3):317–28.

Dealey C. The size of the pressure-sore problem in a teaching hospital. J Adv Nurs 1991 Jun;16(6):663–70.

DeLateur BJ, Berni R, Hangladarom T, Giaconi R. Wheelchair cushions designed to prevent pressure sores: an evaluation. Arch Phys Med Rehabil 1976 Mar;57(3):129–35.

Disa JJ, Carlton JM, Goldberg MH. Efficacy of operative cure in pressure sore patients. Plast Reconstr Surg 1992 Feb;89(2):272–8.

Distel L. More than chart review: a new problem-oriented nursing quality assurance program. QRB Qual Rev Bull 1981 Jan;7(1):26–9.

Dobrzanski S, Kelly CM, Gray JI, Gregg AJ, Cosgrove CA. Granuflex dressings in treatment of full thickness pressure sores. Prof Nurse 1990 Aug;5(11):594–9.

Doughty D, Fairchild P, Stogis S. Your patient: which therapy? J Enterostomal Ther 1990 Jul–Aug;17(4):154–9.

Droessler D, Maibusch RM. Development of a nursing care plan for healing and preventing decubiti. QRB Qual Rev Bull 1979 Aug;5(8):10–14.

Drummond D, Breed AL, Narechania R. Relationship of spine deformity and pelvic obliquity on sitting pressure distributions and decubitus ulceration. J Pediatr Orthop 1985 Jul–Aug;5(4):396–402.

Drummond DS, Narechania RG, Rosenthal AN, Breed AL, Lange TA, Drummond DK. A study of pressure distributions measured during balanced and unbalanced sitting. J Bone Joint Surg Am 1982 Sep;64(7):1034–9.

Ek AC, Boman G. A descriptive study of pressure sores: the prevalence of pressure sores and the characteristics of patients. J Adv Nurs 1982 Jan;7(1):51–7.

Ek AC, Unosson M, Bjurulf P. The modified Norton Scale and the nutritional state. Scand J Caring Sci 1989;3(4):183–7.

El Zayat SG. Preliminary experience with topical phenytoin in wound healing in a war zone. Mil Med 1989 Apr;154(4):178–80.

Engstrand JL. A nursing challenge: effective patient education. AORN J 1979 Sep–Oct;4(5):15–8.

Environmental Protection Agency. Disposal tips for home health care. Washington (DC): U.S. Government Printing Office; 1993 Nov. Report No. EPA530-F-93-027 A. 8 p. Available from: RCRA Docket (5305), U.S. Environmental Protection Agency, 401 M Street, SW, Washington, DC 20460.

Esposito G, Di Caprio G, Ziccardi P, Scuderi N. Tissue expansion in the treatment of pressure ulcers. Plast Reconstr Surg 1991;87(3):501–8. [See Comments in: Plast Reconstr Surg 1991 Dec;88(6):1108, 1116.]

Feedar JA, Kloth LC. Conservative management of chronic wounds. In: Kloth LC, McCulloch JM, Feedar JA, editors. Wound healing: alternatives in management. Philadelphia: FA Davis; 1990.

Feedar JA, Kloth LC, Gentzkow GD. Chronic dermal ulcer healing enhanced with monophasic pulsed electrical stimulation. Phys Ther 1991 Sep;71(9):639–49.

Ferguson-Pell M, Cochran GV, Cardi M, Trachtman L. A knowledge-based program for pressure sore prevention. Ann N Y Acad Sci 1986;463:284–6.

Ferrell BA, Osterweil D, Christenson P. A randomized trial of low-air-loss beds for treatment of pressure ulcers. JAMA 1993 Jan 27;269(4):494–7.

Fincham JE. Smoking cessation: treatment options and the pharmacist's role. Am Pharm 1992 May;NS32(5):62–70.

Firooznia H, Rafii M, Golimbu C, Sokolow J. Computed tomography of pressure sores. J Comput Assist Tomogr 1983a Nov;7(4):367–73.

Firooznia H, Rafii M, Golimbu C, Sokolow J. Computerized tomography in diagnosis of pelvic abscess in spinal-cord-injured patients. Comput Radiol 1983b Nov–Dec;7(6):335–41.

Fisher BH. Topical hyperbaric oxygen treatment of pressure sores and skin ulcers. Lancet 1969;2:405–9.

Fisher J, Arnold PG, Waldorf J, Woods JE. The gluteus maximus musculocutaneous V-Y advancement flap for large sacral defects. Ann Plast Surg 1983 Dec;11(6):517–22.

Fleming A. The action of chemical and physiological antiseptics in a septic wound. Br J Surg 1919;7:99–129.

Foresman PA, Payne DS, Becker D, Lewis D, Rodeheaver GT. A relative toxicity index for wound cleansers. Wounds 1993;5(5):226–31.

Fowler E, Goupil DL. Comparison of the wet-to-dry dressing and a copolymer starch in the management of debrided pressure sores. J Enterostomal Ther 1984 Jan–Feb;11(1):22–5.

French ET, Ledwell-Sifner K. A method for consistent documentation of pressure sores. Rehabil Nurs 1991 Jul–Aug;16(4):204–7.

Freytes HA, Fernandez B, Fleming WC. Ultraviolet light in the treatment of indolent ulcers. South Med J 1965;58:223–6.

Fuhrer MJ, Rintala DH, Hart KA, Clearman R, Young ME. Depressive symptomatology in persons with spinal cord injury who resided in the community. Arch Phys Med Rehabil 1993 Mar;74(3):255–60.

Galpin JE, Chow AW, Bayer AS, Guze LB. Sepsis associated with decubitus ulcers. Am J Med 1976 Sep;61(3):346–50.

Garber SL, Krouskop TA, Carter RE. A system for clinically evaluating wheelchair pressure-relief cushions. Am J Occup Ther 1978 Oct;32(9):565–70.

Garner JS, Favero MS. CDC guidelines for the prevention and control of nosocomial infections: guideline for handwashing and hospital environmental control, 1985. Am J Infect Cont 1986 Jun;14(3):110–29.

Garner JS, Jarvis WR, Emori TG, Horan TC, Hughes JM. CDC definitions for nosocomial infections, 1988. Am J Infect Control 1988 Jun;16(3):128–40 [See Erratum in: Am J Infect Control 1988 Aug;16(4):177.]

Gentzkow GD, Pollack SV, Kloth LC, Stubbs HA. Improved healing of pressure ulcers using dermapulse, a new electrical stimulation device. Wounds 1991 Sep–Oct;3(5):158–70.

Ger R, Levine SA. The management of decubitus ulcers by muscle transposition: an 8-year review. Plast Reconstr Surg 1976 Oct;58(4):419–28.

Gerson LW. The incidence of pressure sores in active treatment hospitals. Int J Nurs Stud 1975;12(4):201–4.

Goren D. Use of Omiderm in treatment of low-degree pressure sores in terminally ill cancer patients. Cancer Nurs 1989 Jun;12(3):165–9.

Gorse GJ, Messner RL. Improved pressure sore healing with hydrocolloid dressings. Arch Dermatol 1987 Jun;123(6):766–71.

Gosnell DJ, Pontius C. A model of quality assurance for decubitus ulcer monitoring. Decubitus 1988 Nov;1(4):24–9.

Gould D. Pressure for change. Nurs Mirror 1985 Oct 16;161(16):28–30.

Gould D. Pressure sore prevention and treatment: an example of nurses' failure to implement research findings. J Adv Nurs 1986 Jul;11(4):389–94.

Gray BC, Salzberg CA, Petro JA, Salisbury RE. The expanded myocutaneous flap for reconstruction of the difficult pressure sore. Decubitus 1990 May;3(2):17–20.

Green E, Katz J. Practice guidelines for management of pressure ulcers. Decubitus 1991 Feb;4(1):36, 38, 40, 42.

Green VA, Carlson HC, Briggs RL, Stewart JL. A comparison of the efficacy of pulsed mechanical lavage with that of rubber-bulb syringe irrigation in removal of debris from avulsive wounds. Oral Surg Oral Med Oral Pathol 1971 Jul;32(1):158–64.

Griffin JW, Tooms RE, Mendius RA, Clifft JK, Vander Zwaag R, El-Zeky F. Efficacy of high voltage pulsed current for healing of pressure ulcers in patients with spinal cord injury. Phys Ther 1991 Jun;71(6):433–42.

Gross A, Cutright DE, Bhaskar SN. Effectiveness of pulsating water jet lavage in treatment of contaminated crushed wounds. Am J Surg 1972 Sep;124(3):373–7.

Gruber RP, Heitkamp DH, Billy LJ, Amato JJ, Arsenal E. Skin permeability of oxygen and hyperbaric oxygen. Arch Surg 1970;101:69–70.

Hackler RH, Zampieri TA. Urethral complications following ischiectomy in spinal cord injury patients: a urethral pressure study. J Urol 1987 Feb;137(2):253–5.

Haher JN, Haher TR, Devlin VJ, Schwartz J. The release of flexion contractures as a prerequisite for the treatment of pressure sores in multiple sclerosis: a report of ten cases. Ann Plast Surg 1983 Sep;11(3):246–9.

Hall PA, Young JV. Autonomic hyperreflexia in spinal cord injured patients: trigger mechanism—dressing changes of pressure sores. J Trauma 1983 Dec;23(12):1074–5.

Haller KB, Reynolds MA, Horsley JA. Developing research-based innovation protocols: process, criteria, and issues. Res Nurs Health 1979 Jun;2(2):45–51.

Hamer ML, Robson MC, Krizek TJ, Southwick WO. Quantitative bacterial analysis of comparative wound irrigations. Ann Surg 1975 Jun;181(6):819–22.

Hamilton L, Quek P, Lew N, Li K, Topp R. Pressure ulcers: an interdisciplinary protocol for prevention and treatment. Perspectives 1989 Spring;13(1):9–15.

Hanan K, Scheele L. Albumin vs. weight as a predictor of nutritional status and pressure ulcer development. Ostomy Wound Manage 1991 Mar–Apr;33(2):22–7.

Hentz VR. Management of pressure sores in a specialty center: a reappraisal. Plast Reconstr Surg 1979 Nov;64(5):683–91.

Hentzen B, Bergstrom N, Pozehl B. Prevalence and incidence of pressure ulcers and associated risk factors in a rural-based home health population. Poster presented at: 17th Annual Midwest Nursing Research Society; 1993 Mar 28–30; Cleveland, OH.

Herceg SJ, Harding RL. Surgical treatment of pressure sores. Arch Phys Med Rehabil 1978 Apr;59(4):193–200.

Heywood AJ, Quaba AA. Modified gluteus maximus V-Y advancement flaps. Br J Plast Surg 1989 May;42(3):263–5.

Hill HL, Brown RG, Jurkiewicz MJ. The transverse lumbosacral back flap. Plast Reconstr Surg 1978;62:177–84.

Hobson DA. Comparative effects of posture on pressure and shear at the body seat interface. J Rehabil Res Dev 1992 Fall;29(4):21–31.

Holman PD. Preservation of the lower extremity in the treatment of massive pressure ulcers. Ariz Med 1985 Feb;42(2):93–9.

Holmes R, Macchiano K, Jhangiani SS, Agarwal NR, Savino JA. Nutrition know-how: combating pressure sores—nutritionally. Am J Nurs 1987 Oct;87(10):1301–3.

Hooker EZ, Sibley P, Nemchausky B, Lopez E. A method for quantifying the area of closed pressure sores by sinography and digitometry. J Neurosci Nurs 1988 Apr;20(2):118–27.

International Association of Enterostomal Therapy. Dermal wounds: pressure sores. Philosophy of the IAET. J Enterostomal Ther 1988 Jan–Feb;15(1):4–17.

Irvine A, Black C. Pressure sore practices. Nurs Times 1990 Sep 19–25;86(38):74–8.

Iverson-Carpenter MS. Focus: nursing diagnosis. Impaired skin integrity. J Gerontol Nurs 1988 Mar;14(3):25–9.

Jackson BS, Chagares R, Nee N, Freeman K. The effects of the Clinitron Bed on pressure ulcers: an experimental study. (Unpublished research report). New York: The Moses Division, Montefiore Medical Center; 1986.

Jackson BS, Chagares R, Nee N, Freeman K. The effects of a therapeutic bed on pressure ulcers: an experimental study. J Enterostomal Ther 1988 Nov–Dec;15(6):220–6.

Jensen TT, Juncker Y. Pressure sores common after hip operations. Acta Orthop Scand 1987 Jun;58(3):209–11.

Johnson AR, White AC, McAnalley B. Comparison of common topical agents for wound treatment: cytotoxicity for human fibroblasts in culture. Wounds 1989 Nov;1(3):186–92.

Johnson CA. Hearing loss following the application of topical neomycin. J Burn Care Rehabil 1988 Mar–Apr;9(2):162–4.

Jones FA. Annual oration on peptic ulcer—in perspective. Trans Med Soc Lond 1985–86;102:101–12.

Jones RC, Shires GT. Principles in the management of wounds. In: Schwartz SI, editor. Principles of surgery. New York: McGraw-Hill; 1974. p. 204.

Kahn J. Case reports: open wound management with the HeNe (6328AU) cold laser. J Orthop Sports Phys Ther 1984;6(3):203–4.

Kaminski MV Jr. Enteral hyperalimentation. Surg Gynecol Obstet 1976 Jul;143(1):12–6.

Karaca AR, Binns JH, Blumenthal FS. Complications of total ischiectomy for the treatment of ischial pressure sores. Plast Reconstr Surg 1978 Jul;62(1):96–9.

Kemp MG, Krouskop TA. Pressure ulcers: reducing the incidence and severity by managing pressure. J Gerontol Nurs 1994;20(9):27–34.

King RB, French ET. Procedures to maintain and restore tissue integrity. In: Rehabilitation Institute of Chicago, Division of Nursing. Rehabilitation nursing procedures manual. Rockville (MD): Aspen; 1990. p. 179–222.

Klein NE, Moore T, Capen D, Green S. Sepsis of the hip in paraplegic patients. J Bone Joint Surg [Am] 1988 Jul;70(6):839–43.

Kloth LC, Feedar JA. Acceleration of wound healing with high voltage, monophasic, pulsed current. Phys Ther 1988 Apr;68(4):503–8. [See Erratum in: Phys Ther 1989 Aug;69(8):702.]

Koshima I, Moriguchi T, Soeda S, Kawata S, Ohta S, Ikeda A. The gluteal perforator-based flap for repair of sacral pressure sores. Plast Reconstr Surg 1993 Apr;91(4):678–83.

Kosiak M. Etiology and pathology of ischemic ulcers. Arch Phys Med Rehabil 1959 Feb;40:62–9.

Krizek TJ, Robson MC. Biology of surgical infection. Surg Clin North Am 1975 Dec;55(6):1261–7.

Kroll SS, Rosenfield L. Perforator-based flaps for low posterior midline defects. Plast Reconstr Surg 1988 Apr;81(4):561–6.

Krouskop TA, Noble PC, Garber SL, Spencer WA. The effectiveness of preventive management in reducing the occurrence of pressure sores. J Rehabil Res Dev 1983 Jul;20(1):74–83.

Krupp S, Kuhn W, Zaech GA. The use of innervated flaps for the closure of ischial pressure sores. Paraplegia 1983 Apr;21(2):119–26.

Kucan JO, Robson MC, Heggers JP, Ko F. Comparison of silver sulfadiazine, povidone-iodine and physiologic saline in the treatment of chronic pressure ulcers. J Am Geriatr Soc 1981 May;29(5):232–5.

Kurzuk-Howard G, Simpson L, Palmieri A. Decubitus ulcer care: a comparative study. West J Nurs Res 1985 Feb;7(1):58–79.

LaMantia JG, Hirschwald JF, Goodman CL, Wooden VM, Delisser O, Staas WE. A program design to reduce chronic readmissions for pressure sores. Rehabil Nurs 1987 Jan–Feb;12(1):22–5.

Langemo DK, Olson B, Hunter S, Burd C, Hansen D, Cathcart-Silberberg T. Incidence of pressure sores in acute care, rehabilitation, extended care, home health, and hospice in one locale. Decubitus 1989 May;2(2):42.

Langemo DK, Olson B, Hunter S, Hansen D, Burd C, Cathcart-Silberberg T. Incidence and prediction of pressure sores in five patient care settings. Decubitus 1991 Aug;4(3):25–6, 28, 30 passim.

Law D. A guide to pressure ulcer prevention care. 1990. Available from: Span America Medical Systems, Inc., Greenville, SC.

Lawton RL, De Pinto V. Bilateral hip disarticulation in paraplegics with decubitus ulcers. Arch Surg 1987 Sep;122(9):1040–3.

Lazarus G, Cooper D, Knighton D, Margolis D, Pecoraro R, Rodeheaver G, Robson M. Definitions and guidelines for assessment of wounds and evaluation of healing. Paper commissioned by the Wound Healing Society, 1992. (Financial support provided by Marion Merrill Dow and Johnson & Johnson). Available from: Wound Healing Society, Richmond, VA.

Lee LK, Ambrus JL. Collagenase therapy for decubitus ulcers. Geriatrics 1975 May;30(5):91–3, 97–8.

Lewis VL Jr. Tensor fasciae latae VY retroposition flap [letter]. Plast Reconstr Surg 1989 Dec;84(6):1016–7.

Lewis VL Jr, Bailey MH, Pulawski G, Kind G, Bashioum RW, Hendrix RW. The diagnosis of osteomyelitis in patients with pressure sores. Plast Reconstr Surg 1988 Feb;81(2):229–32.

Lewis VL Jr, Cunningham BL, Hugo NE. Tensor fasciae latae VY retroposition flap. Ann Plast Surg 1981 Jan;6(1):34–7.

Leyden JJ. Corn starch, Candida albicans, and diaper rash. Pediatr Dermatol 1984 Apr;1(4):322–5.

Leyden JJ, Katz S, Stewart R, Kligman AM. Urinary ammonia and ammonia-producing microorganisms in infants with and without diaper dermatitis. Arch Dermatol 1977 Dec;113(12):1678–80.

Lindan O. Etiology of decubitus ulcers: an experimental study. Arch Phys Med Rehabil 1961 Nov;42(11):774–83.

Lineaweaver W, Howard R, Soucy D, McMorris S, Freeman J, Crain C, Robertson J, Rumley T. Topical antimicrobial toxicity. Arch Surg 1985 Mar;120(3):267–70.

Lingner C, Rolstad BS, Wetherill K, Danielson S. Clinical trial of a moisture vapor-permeable dressing on superficial pressure sores. J Enterostomal Ther 1984 Jul–Aug;11(4):147–9.

Longe RL. Current concepts in clinical therapeutics: pressure sores. Clin Pharm 1986 Aug;5(8):669–81.

Longmire AW, Broom LA, Burch J. Wound infection following high-pressure syringe and needle irrigation [letter]. Am J Emerg Med 1987 Mar;5(2):179–81.

Lubin BS, Powell T. Pressure sores and specialty beds: cost containment and ensurance of quality care. J ET Nurs 1991 Nov–Dec;18(6):190–7.

Luscher NJ, de Roche R, Krupp S, Kuhn W, Zach GA. The sensory tensor fasciae latae flap: a 9-year follow-up. Ann Plast Surg 1991 Apr;26(4):306–10, 311.

Lydon MJ, Hutchinson JJ, Rippon M, Johnson E, de Sousa N, Scudder C, Ryan TJ, Cherry GW. Dissolution of wound coagulum and promotion of granulation tissue under DuoDERM™. Wounds 1989 Aug;1(2):95–106.

Lyman IR, Tenery JH, Basson RP. Correlation between decrease in bacterial load and rate of wound healing. Surg Gynecol Obstet 1970 Apr;130(4):616–21.

Lynch P, Cummings MJ, Roberts PL, Herriott MJ, Yates B, Stamm WE. Implementing and evaluating a system of generic infection precautions: body substance isolation. Am J Infect Control 1990 Feb;18(1):1–12.

Lynch P, Jackson MM, Cummings MJ, Stamm WE. Rethinking the role of isolation practices in the prevention of nosocomial infections. Ann Intern Med 1987 Aug;107(2):243–6.

MacKinnon JL, Cleek PJ. The penetration of ultraviolet light through transparent dressings: a case report. Phys Ther 1984 Feb;64(2):204.

Maklebust J, Magnan MA. Approaches to patient and family education for pressure ulcer management. Decubitus 1992 Jul;5(7):18–20, 24, 26.

Maklebust J, Sieggreen M. Pressure ulcers: guidelines for prevention and nursing management. West Dundee (IL): S-N Publications, 1991. 212 p.

Mandrekas AD, Mastorakos DP. The management of decubitus ulcers by musculocutaneous flaps: a five-year experience. Ann Plast Surg 1992 Feb;28(2):167–74.

Maruyama Y, Hamano Y. Sartorius musculocutaneous flap in the repair of trochanteric pressure sore. Keio J Med 1978 Oct;27(2):63–7.

Maruyama Y, Ohnishi K, Takeuchi S. The lateral thigh fascio-cutaneous flap in the repair of ischial and trochanteric defects. Br J Plast Surg 1984 Jan;37(1):103–7.

Mathes SJ, Feng LJ, Hunt TK. Coverage of the infected wound. Ann Surg 1983 Oct;198(4):420–9.

McDiarmid T, Burns PN, Lewith GT, Machin D. Ultrasound and the treatment of pressure sores. Physiotherapy 1985;71(2):66–70.

McGregor JC, Buchan AC. Our clinical experience with the tensor fasciae latae myocutaneous flap. Br J Plast Surg 1980 Apr;33(2):270–6.

Meehan M. Multisite pressure ulcer prevalence survey. Decubitus 1990 Nov;3(4):14–7.

Melcher RE, Longe RL, Gelbart AO. Pressure sores in the elderly: a systematic approach to management. Postgrad Med 1988 Jan;83(1):299–308.

Merbitz CT, King RB, Bleiberg J, Grip JC. Wheelchair push-ups: measuring pressure relief frequency. Arch Phys Med Rehabil 1985 Jul;66(7):433–8.

Mester E, Mester AF, Mester A. The biomedical effects of laser application. Lasers Surg Med 1985;5(1):31–9.

Micali G, Romeo L. Experience with trapezius and tensor fascia lata myocutaneous flaps. Ann Plast Surg 1982 Aug;9(2):94–100.

Michocki RJ, Lamy PP. The care of decubitus ulcers pressure sores. J Am Geriatr Soc 1976 May;24(5):217–24.

Miller H, Delozier J. Cost implications of the pressure ulcer treatment guideline. Columbia (MD): Center for Health Policy Studies; 1994. Contract No. 282-91-0070. 17 p. Sponsored by the Agency for Health Care Policy and Research.

Miller TV, Rantz M. Quality assurance—guaranteeing a high level of care. J Gerontol Nurs 1989 Nov;15(11):10–5.

Minami RT, Hentz VR, Vistnes LM. Use of vastus lateralis muscle flap for repair of trochanteric pressure sores. Plast Reconstr Surg 1977 Sep;60(3):364–8.

Minami RT, Mills R, Pardoe R. Gluteus maximus myocutaneous flaps for repair of pressure sores. Plast Reconstr Surg 1977 Aug;60(2):242–9.

Moody BL, Fanale JE, Thompson M, Vaillancourt D, Symonds G, Bonasoro C. Impact of staff education on pressure sore development in elderly hospitalized patients. Arch Intern Med 1988 Oct;148(10):2241–3.

Morgan JE. Recurrence of pressure ulcers: a study of five cases. JAMA 1976 Nov 22;236(21):2430–1.

Morison MJ. Pressure sore management: the patient's role. Prof Nurse 1989 Dec;5(3):134, 136, 138 passim.

Motta GJ. The effectiveness of Dermagran topical therapy for treating chronic wounds in nursing facility residents. Ostomy Wound Manage 1991 Sep–Oct;36:35–8.

Muguti GI. Early experience with reconstructive surgery at Mpilo Central Hospital, Zimbabwe. J R Coll Surg Edinb 1990 Aug;35(4):248–51.

Mulder G, Seeley J. The effectiveness of specialty beds in the treatment of severe pressure ulcers in nursing home patients: a preliminary report. (Unpublished research report). Aurora (CO): Wound Healing Institute; 1991.

Mulholland JH, Tui C, Wright AM, Vinci V, Shafiroff B. Protein metabolism and bedsores. Ann Surg 1943;118:1015–23.

Mummery RV, Richardson WW. Clinical trial of Debrisan in superficial ulceration. J Int Med Res 1979;7(4):263–71.

Munro BH, Brown L, Heitman BB. Pressure ulcers: one bed or another? Geriatr Nurs (New York) 1989 Jul–Aug;10(4):190–2.

Nath M, Taylor RG. Ulnar compression neuropathy: an uncommon complication in surgical repair of pressure ulcers. Paraplegia 1978 Feb;16(4):370–4.

National Center for Cost Containment. National specialized bed study and other support surface guidelines. Milwaukee (WI): Department of Veterans Affairs; 1992 Feb. Available from: National Center for Cost Containment, 5000 West National Avenue, Milwaukee, WI 53295.

National Pressure Ulcer Advisory Panel (NPUAP). Pressure ulcers prevalence, cost and risk assessment: consensus development conference statement. Decubitus 1989 May;2(2):24–8.

Neiderhuber S, Stribley R, Koepke G. Reduction of skin bacterial load with use of therapeutic whirlpool. Phys Ther 1975;55(5):482–6.

Neill KM, Conforti C, Kedas A, Burris JF. Pressure sore response to a new hydrocolloid dressing. Wounds 1989 Nov;1(3):173–85.

Nimit K. Public Health Service assessment guidelines for home air-fluidized bed therapy. Health Technol Assess Rep 1989;(5):1–11.

Nuseibeh IM. Split skin graft and the treatment of pressure sores. Paraplegia 1974 May;12(1):1–4.

Nutrition screening manual for professionals caring for older Americans: nutrition screening initiative. Washington (DC): Greer, Margolis, Mitchell, Grunwald & Associates; 1991. 24 p. Available from: The Nutrition Screening Initiative, 2626 Pennsylvania Avenue, NW, Suite 301, Washington, DC 20037.

Oleske DM, Smith XP, White P, Pottage J, Donovan MI. A randomized clinical trial of two dressing methods for the treatment of low-grade pressure ulcers. J Enterostomal Ther 1986 May-Jun;13(3):90-8.

Olsson AG. Intravenous prostacyclin for ischemic ulcers in peripheral artery disease [letter]. Lancet 1980 Nov 15;2(8203):1076.

Oot-Giromini B, Bidwell FC, Heller NB, Parks ML, Prebish EM, Wicks P, Williams PM. Pressure ulcer prevention versus treatment, comparative product cost study. Decubitus 1989 Aug;2(3):52–4.

Paletta CE, Freedman B, Shehadi S. The VY tensor fasciae latae musculocutaneous flap. Plast Reconstr Surg 1989 May;83(5):852–7.

Panel for the Prediction and Prevention of Pressure Ulcers in Adults. Pressure ulcers in adults: prediction and prevention. Clinical Practice Guideline, No. 3. Rockville (MD): Agency for Health Care Policy and Research, Public Health Service, U.S. Department of Health and Human Services; 1992 May. AHCPR Publication No. 92-0047. 63 p.

Parish LC, Witkowski JA. Clinitron therapy and the decubitus ulcer: preliminary dermatologic studies. Int J Dermatol 1980 Nov;19(9):517–8.

Park CA. Activity positioning and ischial tuberosity pressure: a pilot study. Am J Occup Ther 1992 Oct;46(10):904–9.

Parkash S, Banerjee S. The total gluteus maximus rotation and other gluteus maximus musculocutaneous flaps in the treatment of pressure ulcers. Br J Plast Surg 1986 Jan;39(1):66–71.

Parry SW, Mathes SJ. Bilateral gluteus maximus myocutaneous advancement flaps: sacral coverage for ambulatory patients. Ann Plast Surg 1982 Jun;8(6):443–5.

Pearlman NW, McShane RH, Jochimsen PR, Shirazi SS. Hemicorporectomy for intractable decubitus ulcers. Arch Surg 1976 Oct;111(10):1139–43.

Peters W, Cartotto R, Morris S, Jewett M. The rectus femoris myocutaneous flap for closure of difficult wounds of the abdomen, groin, and trochanteric area. Ann Plast Surg 1991 Jun;26(6):572–6.

Petersen NC, Bittmann S. The epidemiology of pressure sores. Scand J Plast Reconstr Surg 1971;5(1)62–6.

Phipps M, Bauman B, Berner D, Butler M, Kalinoski A, Looby M, Malacaria N, Pratt L, Reiley P, Sullivan M. Staging care for pressure sores. Am J Nurs 1984 Aug;84(8):999–1003.

Pinchcofsky-Devin GD, Kaminski MV Jr. Correlation of pressure sores and nutritional status. J Am Geriatr Soc 1986;34(6):435–40.

Powell JW. Increasing acuity of nursing home patients and the prevalence of pressure ulcers: a ten year comparison. Decubitus 1989 May;2(2):56–8.

Putnam T, Calenoff L, Betts HB, Rosen JS. Sinography in management of decubitus ulcers. Arch Phys Med Rehabil 1978 May;59(5):243–5.

Rao DB, Sane PG, Georgiev EL. Collagenase in the treatment of dermal and decubitus ulcers. J Am Geriatr Soc 1975 Jan;23(1):22–30.

Read RC. Presidential address: systemic effects of smoking. Am J Surg 1984 Dec;148(6):706–11.

Reddy NP, Cochran GV. Phenomenological theory underlying pressure-time relationship in decubitus ulcer formation [abstract]. Fed Proc 1979 Mar 1;38(3 Pt 2):1153.

Reichel SM. Shearing force as a factor in decubitus ulcers in paraplegics. JAMA 1958 Feb 15;166(7):762–3.

Relander M, Palmer B. Recurrence of surgically treated pressure sores. Scand J Plast Reconstr Surg Hand Surg 1988;22(1):89–92.

Reuler JB, Cooney TG. The pressure sore: pathophysiology and principles of management. Ann Intern Med 1981 May;94(5):661–6.

Richardson RR, Meyer PR Jr. Prevalence and incidence of pressure sores in acute spinal cord injuries. Paraplegia 1981;19(4):235–47.

Robnett MK. The incidence of skin breakdown in a surgical intensive care unit. J Nurs Qual Assur 1986 Nov;1(1):77–81.

Robson M, Phillips LG, Thomason A, Robson LF, Pierce GF. Recombinant human growth factor-bb for the treatment of chronic pressure ulcers. Ann Plast Surg 1992a;29:193–201.

Robson M, Phillips LG, Thomason A, Robson LF, Pierce GF. Platelet-derived factors BB for treatment of chronic pressure ulcers. Lancet 1992b;339:23–5.

Robson MC. Plastic surgery in quantitative bacteriology: its role in the armamentarium of the surgeon. In: Heggers JP, Robson MC, editors. Boca Raton (FL): CRC Press; 1991. p. 71–84.

Robson MC, Phillips LG, Lawrence WT, Bishop JB, Youngerman JS, Hayward PG, Broemeling LD, Heggers JP. The safety and effect of topically applied recombinant basic fibroblast growth factor on the healing of chronic pressure sores. Ann Surg 1992 Oct;216(4):401–8.

Roche S, Cross S, Burgess I, Pines C, Cayley AC. Cutaneous myiasis in an elderly debilitated patient. Postgrad Med J 1990 Sep;66(779):776–7.

Rodeheaver GT, Kurtz L, Kircher BJ, Edlich RF. Pluronic F-68: a promising new skin wound cleanser. Ann Emerg Med 1980 Nov;9(11):572–6.

Rodeheaver GT, Pettry D, Thacker JG, Edgerton MT, Edlich RF. Wound cleansing by high pressure irrigation. Surg Gynecol Obstet 1975 Sep;141(3):357–62.

Rodeheaver GT, Smith SL, Thacker JG, Edgerton MT, Edlich RF. Mechanical cleansing of contaminated wounds with a surfactant. Am J Surg 1975 Mar;129(3):241–5.

Rosenthal AM, Schurman A. Hyperbaric treatment of pressure sores. Arch Phys Med Rehabil 1971;52:413–3.

Rottkamp B. An experimental nursing study: a behavior modification approach to nursing therapeutics in body position of spinal cord–injured patients. Nurs Res 1976 May–Jun;25(3):181–6.

Rousseau P. Pressure ulcers in an aging society. Wounds 1989 Aug;1(2):135–41.

Royer J, Pickrell K, Georgiade N, Mladick R, Thorne F. Total thigh flaps for extensive decubitus ulcers: a 16 year review of 41 total thigh flaps. Plast Reconstr Surg 1969 Aug;44(2):109–18.

Rubayi S, Cousins S, Valentine WA. Myocutaneous flaps: surgical treatment of severe pressure ulcers. AORN J 1990 Jul;52(1):40–7,50,52–5.

Rubayi S, Pompan D, Garland D. Proximal femoral resection and myocutaneous flap for treatment of pressure ulcers in spinal injury patients. Ann Plast Surg 1991 Aug;27(2):132–8.

Rutala WA. APIC guideline for selection and use of disinfectants. Am J Infect Control 1990 Apr;18(2):99–117.

Rydberg B, Zederfeldt B. Influence of cationic detergents on tensile strength of healing skin wounds in the rat. Acta Chir Scand 1968;134(5):317–20.

Sachs B, Mathews C. Developing a skin care program. Nurs Manage 1990 Aug;21(8):14–5.

Sagi A, Meller Y, Kon M, Rosenberg L, Ben-Yakar Y. Bilateral hip resection for closure of trochanteric pressure sores: case report. Paraplegia 1987 Feb;25(1):39–43.

Salyer J. Wound management in the home: part II. Home Health Nurse 1988 May–Jun;6(3):29–34.

Salzberg CA, Gray BC, Petro JA, Salisbury RE. The perioperative antimicrobial management of pressure ulcers. Decubitus 1990 May;3(2):24–6.

Sanchez S, Eamegdool S, Conway H. Surgical treatment of decubitus ulcers in paraplegics. Plast Reconstr Surg 1969 Jan;43(1):25–8.

Sapico FL, Ginunas VJ, Thornhill-Joynes M, Canawati HN, Capen DA, Klein NE, Khawam S, Montgomerie JZ. Quantitative microbiology of pressure sores in different stages of healing. Diagn Microbiol Infect Dis 1986 May;5(1):31–8.

Saydak SJ. A pilot test of two methods for the treatment of pressure ulcers. J Enterostomal Ther 1990 May–Jun;17(3):139–42.

Schechter JF, Wilkinson RD, Del Carpio J. Anaphylaxis following the use of bacitracin ointment: report of a case and review of the literature. Arch Dermatol 1984 Jul;120(7):909–11.

Scheflan M, Nahai F, Boswick J 3d. Gluteus maximus island musculocutaneous flap for closure of sacral and ischial ulcers. Plast Reconstr Surg 1981 Oct;68(4):533–8.

Schwartz IS, Pervez N. Bacterial endocarditis associated with a permanent transvenous cardiac pacemaker. JAMA 1971 Nov 1;218(5):736–7.

Scott BO. Clinical use of ultraviolet radiation. In: Stillwell GK, editor. Therapeutic electricity and ultraviolet radiation. Baltimore (MD): Williams & Wilkins; 1983. p. 228–62.

Sebern M. Home-team strategies for treating pressure sores. Nursing 1987 Apr;17(4):50–3.

Sebern MD. Pressure ulcer management in home health care: efficacy and cost effectiveness of moisture vapor permeable dressing. Arch Phys Med Rehabil 1986 Oct;67(10):726–9.

Shand JE, McClemont E. Recent advances in the treatment of pressure sores. Paraplegia 1979 Nov;17(4):400–8.

Shannon ML, Skorga P. Pressure ulcer prevalence in two general hospitals. Decubitus 1989 Nov;2(4):38–43.

Shea JD. Pressure sores: classification and management. Clin Orthop 1975 Oct;(112):89–100.

Shetty KR, Duthie EH Jr. Thyrotoxicosis induced by topical iodine application. Arch Intern Med 1990 Nov;150(11):2400–1.

Siddiqui A, Wiedrich T, Lewis V. The tensor fascia lata V-Y retroposition myocutaneous flap: clinical experience. Ann Plast Surg 1993 Mar;30:1–5.

Siegler EL, Lavizzo-Mourey R. Management of stage III pressure ulcers in moderately demented nursing home residents. J Gen Intern Med 1991 Nov–Dec; 6(6):507–13.

Simmons B, Trusler M, Roccaforte J, Smith P, Scott R. Infection control for home health. Infect Control Hosp Epidemiol 1990 Jul;11(7):362–70.

Smoot EC 3d. Clinitron bed therapy hazards [letter]. Plast Reconstr Surg 1986 Jan;77(1):165.

Soriano F, Aguado JM, Tornero J, Fernandez-Guerrero ML, Gomez-Garces JL. Bacteroides fragilis meningitis successfully treated with metronidazole after a previous failure with thiamphenicol. J Clin Microbiol 1986 Sep;24(3):472–3.

Spear SL, Kroll SS, Little JW 3d. Bilateral upper-quadrant (intercostal) flaps: the value of protective sensation in preventing pressure sore recurrence. Plast Reconstr Surg 1987 Nov;80(5):734–6.

St. Clair M. Survey of the uses of the Pegasus airwave system in the United Kingdom. J Tissue Viab 1992;2(1):9–16.

Stevenson TR, Thacker JG, Rodeheaver GT, Bacchetta C, Edgerton MT, Edlich RF. Cleansing the traumatic wound by high pressure syringe irrigation. JACEP 1976 Jan;5(1):17–21.

Stillwell GK. Therapeutic heat and cold. In: Krusen FH, editor. Handbook of physical medicine and rehabilitation. 2nd ed. Philadelphia: Saunders; 1971. p. 259–72.

Strauss MJ, Gong J, Gary BD, Kalsbeek WD, Spear S. The cost of home air-fluidized therapy for pressure sores: a randomized controlled trial. J Fam Pract 1991 Jul;33(1):52–9.

Sugarman B. Osteomyelitis in spinal cord injury. Arch Phys Med Rehabil 1984 Mar;65(3):132–4.

Sugarman B. Pressure sores and underlying bone infection. Arch Intern Med 1987 Mar;147(3):553–5.

Sundell B, Pentti A, Langenskiold A. Surgical treatment of pressure ulcers in paraplegics. Acta Orthop Scand 1967;38(4):532–42.

Surinchak JS, Alago ML, Bellamy RF, Stuck BE, Belkin M. Effects of low-level energy lasers on the healing of full-thickness skin defects. Lasers Surg Med 1983;2(3):267–74.

Taylor TV, Rimmer S, Day B, Butcher J, Dymock IW. Ascorbic acid supplementation in the treatment of pressure sores. Lancet 1974 Sep 7;2(7880):544–6.

Teepe RG, Koebrugge EJ, Lowik CW, Petit PL, Bosboom RW, Twiss IM, Boxma H, Vermeer BJ, Ponec M. Cytotoxic effects of topical antimicrobial and antiseptic agents on human keratinocytes in vitro. J Trauma 1993 Jul;35(1):8–19.

Terz JJ, Schaffner MJ, Goodkin R, Beatty JD, Razor B, Weliky A, Shimabukuro C. Translumbar amputation. Cancer 1990 Jun 15;65(12):2668–75.

Tolhurst DE. "Skin and bone": the use of muscle flaps to cover exposed bone. Br J Plast Surg 1980 Jan;33(1):99–114.

Torrance C. Pressure sores: what goes on? Community Outlook 1983 Nov:332–40.

Tudhope M. Management of pressure ulcers with a hydrocolloid occlusive dressing: results in twenty-three patients. J Enterostomal Ther 1984 May–Jun;11(3):102–5.

University Hospital Consortium. Guidelines for the use of pressure relief devices in the treatment and prevention of pressure ulcers. Oak Brook (IL): University Hospital Consortium Technology Advancement Center; 1990. Available from: University Hospital Consortium Technology Advancement Center, 2001 Spring Road, Suite 700, Oak Brook, IL 60521.

US Preventive Services Task Force. Guide to clinical preventive services: an assessment of the effectiveness of 169 interventions. Baltimore (MD): Williams & Wilkins; 1989. 419 p.

van Rijswijk L. Full-thickness pressure ulcers: patient and wound healing characteristics. Decubitus 1993 Jan;6(1):16–21.

Van Ness CV. The implementation of a quality assurance study and program to reduce the incidence of hospital acquired pressure ulcers. J Enterostomal Ther 1989 Mar–Apr;16(2):61–4.

VanEtten NK, Sexton P, Smith R. Development and implementation of a skin care program. Ostomy Wound Manage 1990 Mar–Apr;27:40–54.

Varma AO, Bugatch E, German FM. Debridement of dermal ulcers with collagenase. Surg Gynecol Obstet 1973 Feb;136(2):281–2.

Vasconez LO, Schneider WJ, Jurkiewicz MJ. Pressure sores. Curr Probl Surg 1977 Apr;14(4):1–62.

Verduin JR, Miller HG, Greer CE. Adults teaching adults. Austin (TX): Learning Concepts; 1977.

Versluysen M. Pressure sores in elderly patients: the epidemiology related to hip operations. J Bone Joint Surg Br 1985 Jan;67(1):10–3.

Versluysen M. How elderly patients with femoral fractures develop pressure sores in hospital. Br Med J Clin Res Ed 1986 May 17;292(6531):1311–3.

Vidal J, Sarrias M. An analysis of the diverse factors concerned with the development of pressure sores in spinal cord patients. Paraplegia 1991 May;29(4):261–7.

Vyas SC, Binns JH, Wilson AN. Thoracolumbar-sacral flaps in the treatment of sacral pressure sores. Plast Reconstr Surg 1980 Feb;65(2):159–63.

Wang TN, Lineaweaver WC, Scott T, Feldman R. Internal pudendal pseudoaneurysm complicating an ischial pressure sore. Ann Plast Surg 1987 Oct;19(4):381–3.

Warner DJ. A clinical comparison of two pressure-reducing surfaces in the management of pressure ulcers. Decubitus 1992 May;5(3):52–5, 58–60, 62–4.

Warren VB, editor. A treasury of techniques for teaching adults. Washington (DC): National Association for Public Continuing and Adult Education; 1977.

Westaby S. Wound care. St. Louis (MO): C. V. Mosby Co.; 1987. p. 14.

Wheeler CB, Rodeheaver GT, Thacker JG, Edgerton MT, Edlich RF. Side-effects of high pressure irrigation. Surg Gynecol Obstet 1976 Nov;143(5):775–8.

Wiersema LA, Lueckenotte AG. Determination of the effectiveness of four sleep surfaces in the treatment of stage 2 and 3 pressure sores. (Unpublished research report). St. Louis (MO): Barnes Hospital; Batesville (IN): Hill-Rom; 1992.

Williams C, Lines C, McKay E. Iron and zinc status in multiple sclerosis patients with pressure sores. Eur J Clin Nutr 1988 Apr;42(4):321–8.

Wills EE, Anderson TW, Beattie BL, Scott A. A randomized placebo-controlled trial of ultraviolet light in the treatment of superficial pressure sores. J Am Geriatr Soc 1983;31(3):131–3.

Xakellis GC, Chrischilles EA. Hydrocolloid versus saline gauze dressings in treating pressure ulcers: a cost-effectiveness analysis. Arch Phys Med Rehabil 1992 May;73:463–9.

Yanai A, Bandoh Y, Tsuzuki K. Bilateral gluteal thigh flaps for closure of large defects in the lumbosacral region and perineal region. Plast Reconstr Surg 1991 Oct;88(4):703–6.

Yarkony GM, Kirk PM, Carlson C, Roth EJ, Lovell L, Heinemann A, King R, Lee MY, Betts HB. Classification of pressure ulcers. Arch Dermatol 1990 Sep;126:1218–9.

Young L. Pressure ulcer prevalence and associated patient characteristics in one long-term care facility. Decubitus 1989 May;2(2):52.

Yuan RT. The use of tissue expansion in lower extremity wounds in paraplegic patients. Plast Reconstr Surg 1989 May;83(5):892–5.

Zimmerer RE, Lawson KD, Calvert CJ. The effects of wearing diapers on skin. Pediatr Dermatol 1986 Feb;3(2):95–101.

Acronyms

AHCPR	Agency for Health Care Policy and Research
APIC	Association for Practitioners in Infection Control
bFGF	Basic fibroblast growth factor
BMI	Body mass index
BSI	Body substance isolation
CDC	Centers for Disease Control and Prevention
CT	Computerized tomography
CURN	Conduct and Utilization of Research in Nursing
DHHS	U.S. Department of Health and Human Services
DMERC	Durable Medical Equipment Regional Carrier
FDA	Food and Drug Administration
IAET	International Association for Enterostomal Therapy
ILD	Indentation load deflection
MRI	Magnetic resonance imaging
MRSA	Methicillin-resistant *Staphylococcus aureus*
NLM	National Library of Medicine
NPC	Nonprotein calories
NPUAP	National Pressure Ulcer Advisory Panel
OBRA	Omnibus Budget Reconciliation Act
OSHA	Occupational Safety and Health Administration
PHS	Public Health Service
psi	pounds per square inch
QI	Quality Improvement
RDA	Recommended daily allowance
rPDGF-BB	Recombinant platelet-derived growth factor-BB

TFL	Tensor fascia lata
TLC	Total lymphocyte count
TPN	Total parenteral nutrition
WBC	White blood count
WOCN	Wound Ostomy and Continence Nurses Society (formerly IAET)

Glossary

Abscess. A circumscribed collection of pus that forms in tissue as a result of acute or chronic localized infection. It is associated with tissue destruction and frequently swelling.

Adherent Materials. Matter attached to the wound bed such as eschar, dirt particles, or bacteria.

Advancing Cellulitis. See Cellulitis.

Air-Flotation Bed. See under Support Surfaces.

Air-Fluidized Bed. See under Support Surfaces.

Alginate Dressing. See under Dressing.

Allergic Sensitization. The development of antibodies to a foreign substance (e.g., medication) that results in an allergic reaction.

Alternating-Air Mattress or Overlay. See under Support Surfaces.

Amyloidosis. A condition characterized by the formation and accumulation of insoluble proteins (amyloid) in various organs of the body, compromising vital function. Amyloid may collect in a chronic wound, such as a pressure ulcer.

Analgesia. Relief of pain without loss of consciousness.

Angular Stomatitis. Single or multiple fissures at the corners of the mouth, one cause of which may be riboflavin deficiency.

Antiseptic (Topical). Product with antimicrobial activity designed for use on skin or other superficial tissues; may damage cells.

Autolytic Debridement. See under Debridement.

Bacteremia. The presence of viable bacteria in the circulating blood.

Bacterial Culture. See Culture (Bacterial).

Bitot's Spots. Superficial, triangular, foamy grey spots on the conjunctiva that consist of keratinized epithelium and are associated with vitamin A deficiency.

Blanchable Erythema. See under Erythema.

Body Substance Isolation (BSI). A system of infection-control procedures routinely used with all patients to prevent cross contamination of pathogens. The system emphasizes the use of barrier precautions to isolate potentially infectious body substances. According to Lynch, Jackson, Cummings, et al. (1987), BSI has six components.

1. Wear gloves for anticipated contact with blood, secretions, mucous membranes, nonintact skin, and moist body substances for all patients. Change gloves before treating another patient. Handwashing between patients is essential.
2. After other types of patient contact, wash the hands for 10 seconds with soap and friction to remove transient microbial flora, and then rinse with running water (Garner and Favero, 1986).
3. Wear additional barriers such as gowns, plastic aprons, masks, or goggles when moist body substances (secretions, blood, or body fluids) are likely to soil the clothing or the skin or splash in the face. The panel notes that protective eyewear, mask (or a faceshield that covers the eyes and face), gloves, and in some cases protective gowns should be used for pressure ulcer irrigation when there is a reasonable expectation that wound secretions might be aerosolized.
4. Place soiled reusable articles and linen, as well as trash, in containers that are securely sealed to prevent leaking. Double bagging is not necessary unless the outside of the bag is visibly soiled.
5. Place needles (without recapping them) and sharp instruments in puncture-resistant, rigid containers. If such containers are not available, recapping using the one-hand technique is acceptable.
6. Assign to private rooms those patients with diseases that could be transmitted by the airborne route (e.g., pulmonary tuberculosis) and other diseases listed under precautions for strict isolation in the category-specific isolation (CDC, 1970). The use of private rooms is also indicated for those patients likely to soil articles in their environment with body substances.

Bottoming Out. Expression used to describe inadequate support from a mattress overlay or seat cushion as determined by a "hand check." To perform a hand check, the caregiver places an outstretched hand (palm up) under the overlay or cushion below the pressure ulcer or that part of the body at risk for a pressure ulcer. If the caregiver feels less than an inch of support material, the patient has bottomed out and the support surface is therefore inadequate.

BSI. See Body Substance Isolation.

Caregiver. Any individual who provides care including professional health care providers, paraprofessional care providers, and family caregivers.

Cellulitis. Inflammation of cellular or connective tissue. Inflammation may be diminished or absent in immunosuppressed individuals.

Cellulitis (Advancing). Cellulitis that is visibly spreading in the area of the wound. Advancement can be monitored by marking the outer edge of the cellulitis and assessing the area for advancement or spread 24 hours later.

Cheilosis. Chapping and fissuring of the lips, which may be caused by vitamin B_2 deficiency.

Chemical Debridement. See under Debridement.

Clean. Containing no foreign material or debris.

Clean Dressing. Dressing that is not sterile but is free of environmental contaminants such as water damage, dust, pest and rodent contaminants, and gross soiling. See Chapter 5 for the specific measures necessary to keep dressings clean.

Clean Wound. Wound free of purulent drainage, devitalized tissue, or dirt.

Colonized. The presence of bacteria on the surface or in the tissue of a wound without indications of infection such as purulent exudate, foul odor, or surrounding inflammation. All Stage II, III, and IV pressure ulcers are colonized.

Contaminated. Containing bacteria, other microorganisms, or foreign material. The term usually refers to bacterial contamination and in this context is synonymous with colonized. Wounds with bacterial counts of 10^5 organisms per gram of tissue or less are generally considered contaminated; those with higher counts are generally considered infected.

Continuously Moist Saline Gauze. See under Dressing.

Culture (Bacterial). Removal of bacteria from a wound for the purpose of placing them in a growth medium in the laboratory to propagate to the point where they can be identified and tested for sensitivity to various antibiotics. Swab cultures are generally inadequate for this purpose.

Culture (Quantitative Bacterial). Performing a bacterial culture in a manner that allows the number of bacteria present in a known quantity of tissue biopsy, wound aspirate, or sampled surface to be quantified.

Culture and Sensitivity. Removal of bacteria from a wound for the purpose of placing them in a growth medium in the laboratory to propagate to the point where they can be identified and tested for sensitivity to various antibiotics.

Culture (Swab). Technique involving the use of a swab to remove bacteria from a wound and place them in a growth medium for propagation and identification. Swab cultures obtained from the surface of a pressure ulcer are usually positive because of surface colonization and should not be used to diagnose ulcer infection.

Cytotoxic Cleansers. Agents that can be used to cleanse wounds (to remove undesirable materials) but that have a specific destructive action on certain cells.

Dakin's® Solution. Buffered sodium hypochlorite; a bactericidal wound irrigant.

Dead Space. A cavity remaining in a wound.

Debridement. Removal of devitalized tissue and foreign matter from a wound. Various methods can be used for this purpose:

> **Autolytic Debridement.** The use of synthetic dressings to cover a wound and allow eschar to self-digest by the action of enzymes present in wound fluids.
>
> **Enzymatic (Chemical) Debridement.** The topical application of proteolytic substances (enzymes) to breakdown devitalized tissue.
>
> **Mechanical Debridement.** Removal of foreign material and devitalized or contaminated tissue from a wound by physical forces rather than by chemical (enzymatic) or natural (autolytic) forces. Examples are wet-to-dry dressings, wound irrigation, whirlpool, and dextranomers.
>
> **Sharp Debridement.** Removal of foreign material or devitalized tissue by a sharp instrument such as a scalpel. Laser debridement is also considered a type of sharp debridement.

Decubitus Ulcer. See Pressure Ulcer.

Dehiscence. Separation of the layers of a surgical wound.

Delay of Flaps. See under Operative Repair.

Deterioration. Negative course. Failure of the pressure ulcer to heal, as shown by wound enlargement that is not brought about by debridement.

Dextranomers. Highly hydrophilic dextran-polymer beads that are poured into secreting wounds to absorb wound exudates and act as a debriding agent.

Devitalized Tissue. See Necrotic Tissue.

Direct Closure. See under Operative Repair.

Disinfection. A process that eliminates many or all pathogenic microorganisms on inanimate objects, with the exception of bacterial spores. Disinfection of pressure ulcers is neither desirable nor feasible.

Donut-Type Device. See under Support Surfaces.

Dressing. The material applied to a wound for the protection of the wound and absorbance of drainage.

Alginate Dressing. A nonwoven absorptive dressing manufactured from seaweed.

Film Dressing. A clear, adherent, nonabsorptive, polymer-based dressing that is permeable to oxygen and water vapor but not to water.

Foam Dressing. A spongelike polymer dressing that may or may not be adherent; it may be impregnated or coated with other materials and has some absorptive properties.

Gauze Dressing. A cotton or synthetic fabric dressing that is absorptive and permeable to water, water vapor, and oxygen. This dressing may be impregnated with petrolatum, antiseptics, or other agents.

Wet-to-Dry Saline Gauze. A dressing technique in which gauze moistened with normal saline is applied wet to the wound and removed once the gauze becomes dry and adheres to the wound bed. The goal is to debride the wound as the dressing is removed.

Continuously Moist Saline Gauze. A dressing technique in which gauze moistened with normal saline is applied to the wound and remoistened frequently enough so it will remain moist. The goal is to maintain a continuously moist wound environment.

Hydrocolloid Dressing. An adhesive, moldable wafer made of a carbohydrate-based material, usually with a waterproof backing. This dressing usually is impermeable to oxygen, water, and water vapor and has some absorptive properties.

Hydrogel Dressing. A water-based, nonadherent, polymer-based dressing that has some absorptive properties.

Pastes/Powders/Beads. Agents formulated primarily to fill wound cavities that may have some absorptive properties.

Dynamic Device. See under Support Surfaces.

Electrical Stimulation. The use of an electrical current to transfer energy to a wound. The type of electricity that is transferred is controlled by the electrical source.

Endocarditis. Inflammation of the innermost tunic of the heart, which includes the endothelium and subendothelial connective tissue.

Epithelialization. The stage of tissue healing in which the epithelial cells migrate (move) across the surface of a wound. During this stage of healing, the epithelium appears the color of "ground glass" to pink.

Erythema. Redness of the skin.

> **Blanchable Erythema.** Reddened area that temporarily turns white or pale when pressure is applied with a fingertip. Blanchable erythema over a pressure site is usually due to a normal reactive hyperemic response.
>
> **Nonblanchable Erythema.** Redness that persists when fingertip pressure is applied. Nonblanchable erythema over a pressure site is a symptom of a Stage I pressure ulcer.

Eschar. Thick, leathery, necrotic, devitalized tissue.

Exudate. Any fluid that has been extruded from a tissue or its capillaries, more specifically because of injury or inflammation. It is characteristically high in protein and white blood cells.

Fascia. A sheet or band of fibrous tissue that lies deep below the skin or encloses muscles and various organs of the body.

Film Dressing. See under Dressing.

Fluctuance. Wavelike motion, indicative of the presence of fluid, used to describe the appearance of wound tissue.

Fluid Irrigation. Cleansing by means of a stream of fluid, preferably saline.

Foam Dressing. See under Dressing.

Foam Mattress Overlay. See under Support Surfaces.

Free Flap. See under Operative Repair.

Friction. Mechanical force exerted when skin is dragged across a coarse surface such as bed linens.

Full Thickness Tissue Loss. The absence of epidermis and dermis.

Gauze Dressing. See under Dressing.

Glossitis. Inflammation of the tongue, which may be due to multiple B-vitamin deficiencies.

Granulation Tissue. The pink/red, moist tissue that contains new blood vessels, collagen, fibroblasts, and inflammatory cells, which fills an open, previously deep wound when it starts to heal.

Growth Factors. Proteins that affect the proliferation, movement, maturation, and biosynthetic activity of cells. For the purposes of this guideline, these are proteins that can be produced by living cells.

Hand Check. A method of checking whether a patient is "bottoming out." See Bottoming Out.

Handwashing. Handwashing is the cornerstone of any infection-control program. Handwashing should be of sufficient duration to remove the transient microbial flora (10 seconds of soap and friction, followed by rinsing with running water).

Healing. A dynamic process in which anatomical and functional integrity is restored. This process can be monitored and measured. For wounds of the skin, it involves repair of the dermis (granulation tissue formation) and epidermis (epithelialization). Healed wounds represent a spectrum of repair: They can be ideally healed (tissue regeneration), minimally healed (temporary return of anatomical continuity), or acceptably healed (sustained functional and anatomical result). The acceptably healed wound is the ultimate outcome of wound healing but not necessarily the appropriate outcome for all patients.

Primary Intention Healing. Closure and healing of a sutured wound.

Secondary Intention Healing. Closure and healing of a wound by the formation of granulation tissue and epithelialization.

Heterotopic Bone Formation. Growth of bone at an abnormal site on the body. Such growth may be a complication of pressure ulcers.

Hydrocolloid Dressing. See under Dressing.

Hydrogel Dressing. See under Dressing.

Hydrotherapy. Use of whirlpool or submersion in water for wound cleansing.

Hyperbaric Oxygen. Oxygen at greater than atmospheric pressure that can be applied either to the whole patient inside a pressurized chamber or to a localized area (such as an arm or leg) inside a smaller chamber.

Hypoalbuminemia. An abnormally low amount of albumin in the blood. A value less than 3.5 mg/dL is clinically significant. Albumin is the major serum protein that maintains plasma colloidal osmotic pressure (pressure within blood vessels) and transports fatty acids, bilirubin, and many drugs as well as certain hormones, such as cortisol and thyroxine, through the blood. Low serum albumin may be due to inadequate protein intake, active inflammation, or serious hepatic and renal disease and is associated with pressure ulcer development.

Incidence. Rate at which new cases of a condition occur during a specific time period.

Infection. The presence of bacteria or other microorganisms in sufficient quantity to damage tissue or impair healing. Clinical experience has indicated that wounds can be classified as infected when the wound tissue contains 10^5 or greater microorganisms per gram of tissue. Clinical signs of infection may not be present, especially in the immunocompromised patient or the patient with a chronic wound.

Infection (Clinical). The presence of bacteria or other microorganisms in sufficient quantity to overwhelm the tissue defenses and produce the inflammatory signs of infection—i.e., purulent exudate, odor, erythema, warmth, tenderness, edema, pain, fever, and elevated white cell count.

> **Local Clinical Infection.** A clinical infection that is confined to the wound and within a few millimeters of its margins.
>
> **Systemic Clinical Infection.** A clinical infection that extends beyond the margins of the wound. Some systemic infectious complications of pressure ulcers include cellulitis, advancing cellulitis, osteomyelitis, meningitis, endocarditis, septic arthritis, bacteremia, and sepsis. See Sepsis.

Inflammatory Response. A localized protective response elicited by injury or destruction of tissues that serves to destroy, dilute, or wall off both the injurious agent and the injured tissue. Clinical signs include pain, heat, redness, swelling, and loss of function. Inflammation may be diminished or absent in immunosuppressed patients.

Innervation. Nerve supply to an area of the body. Innervation is considered adequate if it is sufficient to sense temperature, touch, and pressure/pain and communicate this sensory information to the brain.

Interface Pressure. See Pressure (Interface).

Irrigation. Cleansing by a stream of fluid, preferably saline.

Ischemia. Deficiency of blood supply to a tissue, often leading to tissue necrosis.

Local Clinical Infection. See under Infection (Clinical).

Low-Air-Loss Bed. See under Support Surfaces.

Macerate. To soften by wetting or soaking. In this context it refers to degenerative changes and disintegration of skin when it has been kept too moist.

Malnutrition. State of nutritional insufficiency due to either inadequate dietary intake or defective assimilation or utilization of food ingested.

Clinically significant malnutrition is diagnosed if (1) serum albumin is less than 3.5 mg/dL, (2) the total lymphocyte count is less than 1,800/mm^3, or (3) body weight has decreased more than 15 percent.

Mattress Replacement System. See under Support Surfaces.

Mechanical Debridement. See under Debridement.

Mechanical Loading. The contribution of mechanical forces—i.e., pressure, friction, and shear—to the development of pressure ulcers.

Meningitis. Inflammation of the membranes of the brain or spinal cord.

Moist Saline Gauze. See under Dressing.

Moisture. In the context of this document, moisture refers to skin moisture that may increase the risk of pressure ulcer development and impair healing of existing ulcers. Primary sources of skin moisture include perspiration, urine, feces, drainage from wounds, or fistulas.

Muscle Flap. See under Operative Repair.

Musculocutaneous Flap. See under Operative Repair.

Necrosis. Death of tissue.

Necrotic Tissue. Tissue that has died and has therefore lost its usual physical properties and biological activity. Also called "devitalized tissue."

Needle Aspiration. Removal of fluid from a cavity by suction, often to obtain a sample (aspirate) for culturing.

Nonblanchable Erythema. See under Erythema.

No-Touch Technique. Method of changing surface dressings without touching the wound or the surface of any dressing that may be in contact with the wound. Adherent dressings should be grasped by the corner and removed slowly, whereas gauze dressings can be pinched in the center and lifted off.

Operative Repair. In the context of this guideline, operative repair refers to a variety of surgical procedures designed to repair the pressure ulcer.

> **Delay of Flaps.** The development and transfer of a flap to a recipient site in more than one step to ensure its vascular supply.
>
> **Direct Closure.** Direct primary closure with sutures. This approach stretches the skin and creates tension that frequently leads to dehiscence and therefore is seldom used except for small, superficial ulcers.
>
> **Free Flap.** A procedure involving a muscle-type flap in which the vein and artery are disconnected at the donor site and reconnected to the vessels at the recipient site with the aid of a microscope.

Muscle Flap. A procedure that moves a known muscle along with its vascular supply (either intact or reestablished) into a defect.

Musculocutaneous Flap. A procedure that moves muscle combined with a portion of overlying skin having an intact vascular supply. The portion of skin overlying the muscle is fed by perforators within the muscle. This type of flap has several advantages: It is fed by named, identifiable blood vessels; supplies higher concentrations of oxygen to underlying bone, which may help heal osteomyelitis; can limit the effects of shear and ulcer recurrence; and provides more bulk, which may limit the effect of ischemia. However, muscle tolerates warm ischemia less well than skin.

Sensate Flap. A procedure that moves muscle, skin, and a sensory nerve. The sensory nerve provides feeling to the flap.

Skin Flap. A procedure that moves a section of skin and associated subcutaneous tissue from one part of the body to another, with the vascular supply maintained for nourishment. The vascular attachment can be the original vessel, rotated along with the flap; changed from one part of the flap to another; or reestablished by microvascular anastomoses once it has been placed in the new location. One disadvantage of local flap closure is that the flap essentially redistributes an already inadequately perfused tissue and is randomly dependent on an unpredictable local blood supply.

Skin Graft. A procedure that moves a segment of dermis and a portion of epidermis. The graft is completely separated from its blood supply and donor site and moved to a recipient site. Skin grafts contain varying portions of epidermis and dermis and can be full thickness or partial thickness, depending upon how much dermis is included in the graft. One disadvantage of skin grafts applied to granulating bone is that there is no padding and they quickly erode.

Tissue Expansion. A surgical technique during which an expandable device is placed beneath viable skin. The device is expanded with serial injections of saline and when the skin has stretched, it is moved to cover a nearby defect.

V-Y Advancement. This procedure derives its name from the appearance of the postoperative wound. After an incision is made in the shape of a "V," the apex of the "V" is closed by advancing the central portion. This leaves a scar that looks like a "Y."

Osteomyelitis. Inflammation of the bone marrow and adjacent bone, often due to infection.

Overlay. See under Support Surfaces.

Pastes/Powders/Beads. See under Dressing.

Perineal–Urethral Fistula. An abnormal passageway between the perineum (area between the scrotum or vulva and the anus) and the urethra (canal conveying urine from the bladder to the exterior of the body). Such a fistula may be a complication of pressure ulcer(s).

Phagocytic Demand. The amount of particulate material (such as bacteria) that white blood cells must ingest in an area.

Phagocytosis. The process of ingestion and digestion of bacteria, cells, necrotic tissue, or debris by white blood cells in an injured area.

Polypharmacy. The administration of many drugs concurrently, usually meaning that a patient is receiving an excessive number of medications. Polypharmacy may negatively affect adherence to the pressure ulcer treatment plan.

Pressure (Interface). Force per unit area that acts perpendicularly between the body and the support surface. This parameter is affected by the stiffness of the support surface, the composition of the body tissue, and the geometry of the body being supported.

Pressure Reduction. Reduction of interface pressure, not necessarily below the level required to close capillaries (i.e., capillary-closing pressure).

Pressure Relief. Reduction of interface pressure below capillary-closing pressure.

Pressure Ulcer. Any lesion caused by unrelieved pressure resulting in damage of underlying tissue. Also called decubitus ulcer, pressure sore, and bed sore. Pressure ulcers are usually located over bony prominences and are graded or staged to classify the degree of tissue damage observed. Such staging is used as a tool for communication and assessment. The recommendations regarding staging put forth by this panel are consistent with those of the National Pressure Ulcer Advisory Panel Consensus Development Conference (NPUAP, 1989), as derived from previous staging systems proposed by Shea (1975) and the Wound Ostomy and Continence Nurses Society (WOCN). Numerical identification of stages does not necessarily imply a progression in ulcer severity. For example, a Stage I ulcer may have very little tissue damage or it may have necrotic underlying tissue, because muscle tissue is more sensitive than skin to pressure-induced ischemia. Pressure ulcers are staged as follows:

Stage I. Nonblanchable erythema of intact skin, the heralding lesion of skin ulceration. In individuals with darker skin, discoloration of the skin, warmth, edema, induration, or hardness may also be indicators.

Stage II. Partial thickness skin loss involving epidermis, dermis, or both. The ulcer is superficial and presents clinically as an abrasion, blister, or shallow crater.

Stage III. Full thickness skin loss involving damage to or necrosis of subcutaneous tissue that may extend down to, but not through, underlying fascia. The ulcer presents clinically as a deep crater with or without undermining of adjacent tissue.

Stage IV. Full thickness skin loss with extensive destruction, tissue necrosis, or damage to muscle, bone, or supporting structures (e.g., tendon, joint capsule). Undermining and sinus tracts may also be associated with Stage IV pressure ulcers.

The following limitations are inherent in these definitions:

1. Because the skin remains intact in Stage I pressure ulcers, these lesions are not ulcers in the usual sense. In addition, Stage I pressure ulcers are not always reliably assessed, especially in patients with darkly pigmented skin. A reliable system to accurately identify Stage I pressure ulcers in individuals with darkly pigmented skin should be developed. Despite these limitations, identification of a Stage I pressure ulcer is critical for indicating the need for more vigilant assessment and preventive care.
2. When eschar is present, a pressure ulcer cannot be accurately staged until the eschar has been removed.
3. It may be difficult to assess pressure ulcers in patients with casts, other orthopedic devices, or support stockings. Routine assessment to check for adequate circulation, movement, and sensation may fail to detect pressure ulcers beneath casts. Health care providers should (1) assess the skin under the edges of casts, (2) be alert to patient complaints of pressure-induced pain, (3) determine whether casts need to be altered or replaced to relieve pressure, and (4) remove support stockings to assess the skin.

Prevalence. The number of cases present in a population at one point in time.

Primary Intention Healing. See under Healing.

Pseudoaneurysm. Dilatation and tortuosity of a blood vessel, a potential complication of pressure ulcers.

psi. Pounds per square inch—a unit of pressure, in this case, the pressure exerted by a stream of fluid against one square inch of skin or wound surface.

Purulent Discharge/Drainage. A product of inflammation that contains pus—i.e., cells (leukocytes, bacteria) and liquefied necrotic debris.

Qualitative Data. Information that describes the nature or qualities of a subject.

Quantitative Bacterial Culture. See Culture.

Quantitative Data. Information that describes the characteristics of a subject in numerical or quantitative terms.

Reactive Hyperemia. Reddening of the skin caused by blood rushing back into ischemic tissue.

Repositioning. Any change in body position that relieves pressure from tissue overlying bony prominences. Periodic repositioning of chairbound and bedfast individuals is one of the most basic and frequently used methods of reducing pressure. The overall goal of repositioning is to allow tissue reperfusion and thus prevent ischemic tissue changes. The term "repositioning" implies a sustained relief of pressure, not just a temporary shift. Specific repositioning techniques and the frequency of repositioning should be individualized according to the patient's level of risk and the goals of care.

Saline Gauze. See under Dressing.

Secondary Intention Healing. See under Healing.

Sensate Flap. See under Operative Repair.

Sepsis. The presence of various pus-forming and other pathogenic organisms or their toxins, in the blood or tissues. Clinical signs of blood-borne sepsis include fever, tachycardia, hypotension, leukocytosis, and a deterioration in mental status. The same organism is often isolated in both the blood and the pressure ulcer.

Septic Arthritis. Inflammation of joints caused by bacterial invasion, a potential complication of pressure ulcers.

Seroma. A collection of serum/plasma within a wound.

Sharp Debridement. See under Debridement.

Shear. Mechanical force that acts on a unit area of skin in a direction parallel to the body's surface. Shear is affected by the amount of pressure exerted, the coefficient of friction between the materials contacting each other, and the extent to which the body makes contact with the support surface.

Sinus Tract. A cavity or channel underlying a wound that involves an area larger than the visible surface of the wound.

Skin Equivalent. A material used to cover open tissue that acts as a substitute for nascent (beginning) dermis and epidermis and that has at least some of the characteristics of human skin (e.g., amniotic tissue, xenografts, human allografts). For the purpose of this guideline, only tissue with viable, biologically active cells is given this designation.

Skin Flap. See under Operative Repair.

Skin Graft. See under Operative Repair.

Slough. Necrotic (dead) tissue in the process of separating from viable portions of the body.

Squamous Cell Carcinoma. A malignant new growth that arises from epithelial cells and has a cuboid appearance. When arising within a chronic ulcer, it is commonly referred to as Marjolin's ulcer.

Stasis Ulcer. Ulceration associated with ambulatory venous hypertension.

Static Air Mattress. See under Support Surfaces.

Static Device. See under Support Surfaces.

Static Support Surface. See under Support Surfaces.

Static Water Mattress. See under Support Surfaces.

Stratum Corneum. Outermost layer of the epidermis.

Support Surfaces. Special beds, mattresses, mattress overlays, or seat cushions that reduce or relieve pressure while sitting or lying.

Air-Flotation Bed. Generic descriptor for low-air-loss beds and air-fluidized beds.

Air-Fluidized Bed. Class of support surfaces that uses a high rate of air flow to fluidize fine particulate material (such as sand) to produce a support medium that has characteristics similar to a liquid.

Alternating-Air Mattress or Overlay. Mattress or overlay with interconnecting air cells that cyclically inflate and deflate to produce alternating high and low pressure intervals. Cells with larger depth and diameter produce greater pressure relief over the body.

Donut-Type Device. A rigid, ring-shaped device created to relieve pressure on the sitting surface. This device is not recommended, because even though pressure is relieved in the tissue over the center of the ring, pressure in tissue resting on the ring causes vascular congestion and may impede circulation to the tissues.

Dynamic Device (or Dynamic Support Surface). Pressure-reducing device designed to change its support characteristics in a cyclical fashion. Examples include alternating-air mattresses and mechanical seats that change shape and redistribute pressure.

Foam Mattress Overlay. Thick foam slab with a textured surface designed to be placed on top of the standard hospital mattress to reduce pressure by enveloping the body. Its effectiveness is influenced by its thickness, density, and stiffness.

Low-Air-Loss Bed. A series of interconnected woven fabric air pillows that allow some air to escape through the support surface. The pillows can be variably inflated to adjust the level of pressure relief.

Mattress Replacement System. Mattress with pressure-reducing or pressure-relieving features that can be placed on an existing bed frame.

Overlay. General term used to describe support surfaces placed on top of a standard hospital mattress.

Static Air Mattress. A vinyl mattress overlay composed of interconnected air cells that are inflated with a blower before use. The shifting of air among the cells distributes pressure uniformly over the support area to create a flotation effect.

Static Device (or Static Support Surface). Pressure-reducing device designed to provide support characteristics that remain constant—i.e., do not cycle in time. Examples include foam overlays, cushions, and water mattresses.

Static Water Mattress. A vinyl mattress or overlay composed of interconnected compartments that are filled with water to distribute pressure uniformly over the support surface to create a flotation effect.

Surfactants. A surface-active agent that reduces the surface tension of fluids to allow greater penetration.

Swab Culture. See Culture (Swab).

Systemic Clinical Infection. See under Infection (Clinical).

Tissue Biopsy. Use of a sharp instrument to obtain a sample of skin, muscle, or bone.

Tissue Expansion. See under Operative Repair.

Tissue Load. The distribution of pressure, friction, and shear on tissue.

Topical Antibiotic. A drug known to inhibit or kill microorganisms that can be applied locally to a tissue surface.

Topical Antiseptic. Product with antimicrobial activity designed for use on skin or other superficial tissues; may damage some cells.

Trochanter. Bony prominence on the upper part of the femur.

Tunneling. A passageway under the surface of the skin that is generally open at the skin level; however, most of the tunneling is not visible.

Underlying Tissue. Tissue that lies beneath the surface of the skin such as fatty tissue, supporting structures, muscle, and bone.

Undermining. A closed passageway under the surface of the skin that is open only at the skin surface. Generally it appears as an area of skin ulceration at the margins of the ulcer with skin overlying the area. Undermining often develops from shearing forces.

V-Y Advancement. See under Operative Repair.

Wet-to-Dry Saline Gauze. See under Dressing.

Wound Healing. See Healing.

Contributors

This section acknowledges the numerous individuals and organizations that contributed their time and expertise to the development of this guideline. Contributors include panel members, consultants, panel staff, editorial staff, library services, contractor support personnel, AHCPR personnel, individual peer reviewers, and pilot site reviewers. Without their intense efforts and collaborative endeavors, this guideline would not have been possible.

Treatment of Pressure Ulcers Guideline Panel

Nancy Bergstrom, PhD, RN, FAAN, *Chair*
Professor and Interim Associate Dean
Graduate Nursing Programs
University of Nebraska Medical Center
Omaha, Nebraska
Dr. Bergstrom is actively engaged in research on nutrition and the etiology of pressure ulcers and has been instrumental in the testing and further development of the Braden Scale for Predicting Pressure Sore Risk. She is President of the Midwest Nursing Research Society and past Chair of the American Nurses Association's Council of Nurse Researchers. She has written numerous articles, served as a peer reviewer, and received support in her research efforts by the National Institutes of Health. She is the recipient of the first Kosiak Award presented by the National Pressure Ulcer Advisory Panel in 1991; the American Nurses Association's Jessie M. Scott Award for demonstrating the interdependence of nursing education, nursing practice, and nursing research; and the Baxter Foundation Episteme Award from Sigma Theta Tau International for her leadership in developing the pressure ulcer prevention guideline.

Richard M. Allman, MD
Associate Professor of Medicine
Director of the Center for Aging and the Division of Gerontology and Geriatrics
University of Alabama at Birmingham
Chief of Geriatrics Section, Birmingham Department of Veterans Affairs Medical Center
Birmingham, Alabama
Dr. Allman is actively involved in studies of different topical agents for pressure ulcers, pressure ulcer risk factors, and the implications of pressure ulcers on health care costs, morbidity, and mortality. He serves as a vice-president of the National Pressure Ulcer Advisory Panel and on the Councils of the American Federation for Clinical Research and the Association of

Directors of Geriatric Academic Programs. He serves on the editorial boards of the *Journal of the American Geriatrics Society* and *Advances in Wound Care*. Dr. Allman's research on pressure ulcers has been published in the *New England Journal of Medicine* and the *Annals of Internal Medicine*, and he has contributed chapters to multiple textbooks of geriatric medicine and Kelly's *Textbook of Internal Medicine*.

Oscar M. Alvarez, PhD
Director of the University Wound Healing Clinic
New Brunswick, New Jersey
Dr. Alvarez received his doctorate in biochemistry from Rutgers University and his medical training from the University of Madrid, Madrid, Spain. He has been the recipient of many research grants and awards to study wound healing. Dr. Alvarez has held faculty positions with the University of Pittsburgh School of Medicine, Cornell University Medical College, and Rockefeller University. Currently, Dr. Alvarez is the Director of the University Wound Healing Clinic and is a part-time faculty member at the University of Medicine and Dentistry of New Jersey. Dr. Alvarez serves on the editorial board of the journal *Wounds* and is the author of more than 80 major publications on the subject of wound care and pressure ulcer management.

M. Alisan Bennett, EdD, RN
Supervisor and Special Projects Coordinator, Nursing Education and Research
Woodhull Medical and Mental Health Center of the New York City Health and Hospitals Corporation
Brooklyn, New York
Dr. Bennett is active in clinical research related to nursing practice and education, with emphasis on public health and cultural diversity. She has published and presented on the topic of early detection and prevention of pressure ulcers in persons with darkly pigmented, intact skin. A member of the British Society for Tissue Viability, she consults annually with clinical nurse researchers in London, England, regarding the detection and treatment of pressure ulcers. She has conducted research on the interdisciplinary management of pressure ulcers at the Royal College of Nursing and the Royal Society of Nursing.

Carolyn E. Carlson, PhD, RN
Professor of Nursing, Cedarville College
Cedarville, Ohio
Associate Director of Nursing and Allied Health for Research and Evaluation, Division of Nursing and Allied Health, and Department of Research, Rehabilitation Institute of Chicago
Chicago, Illinois

Dr. Carlson is principal investigator of a program grant, "Prevention of Pressure Sores after Spinal Cord Injury," and coprincipal investigator of "Adaptation After Stroke: Patient and Primary Support Person," funded by the National Institute for Nursing Research. Dr. Carlson is coauthor of "Skin Integrity" in the *Annual Review of Nursing Research* and is on the editorial board of *Topics in Geriatric Rehabilitation.*

Rita A. Frantz, PhD, RN, FAAN
Associate Professor, College of Nursing
University of Iowa
Clinical Associate in Nursing
Iowa Veterans Home
Iowa City, Iowa

Dr. Frantz has studied biophysical factors in pressure ulcer development. She is now conducting a multicenter clinical trial to evaluate the efficacy of transcutaneous electrical nerve stimulation on healing of recalcitrant pressure ulcers. Dr. Frantz currently serves as a consultant on pressure ulcers and wound management to several long-term care facilities and was formerly a consultant to the Priority Expert Panel on Long-Term Care for Older Adults at the National Center for Nursing Research.

Susan L. Garber, MA, OTR, FAOTA
Assistant Director for Research and Education, Department of Occupational Therapy
The Institute for Rehabilitation and Research
Assistant Professor, Department of Physical Medicine and Rehabilitation
Baylor College of Medicine
Houston, Texas

Mrs. Garber is an occupational therapist who has participated in pressure ulcer research since 1975, often as principal investigator or coinvestigator. She has published on the topic of pressure ulcers in both peer-reviewed journals and books and serves as a reviewer for the *American Journal of Occupational Therapy* and the *Archives of Physical Medicine and Rehabilitation*. In addition, Mrs. Garber serves on the board of the Texas Occupational Therapy Association, Gulf Coast East District.

Bettie S. Jackson, EdD, MBA, FAAN
Director of Professional Services, Department of Nursing
Moses Division, Montefiore Medical Center
Bronx, New York
Associate Research Scientist, School of Nursing, Columbia University
New York, New York
Dr. Jackson is coeditor of the textbook *Principles of Ostomy Care* and is an Enterostomal Therapy Nurse. She has published more than 65 papers, is book review editor for *The American Journal of Critical Care*, and serves on the editorial boards of *Journal of Nursing Administration* and *Cancer Nursing*. She is a former president of the International Association for Enterostomal Therapy. Dr. Jackson is a Fellow in the National Academies of Practice.

Mitchell V. Kaminski, Jr., MD, SC, FACS, FICS, FACN
Staff Surgeon, Thorek Hospital and Medical Center
Clinical Professor of Surgery, Chicago Medical School
University of Health Sciences
Chicago, Illinois
Dr. Kaminski is a Diplomate, American Boards of Surgery and Nutrition. He is also in private practice and actively involved in clinical research. One research focus has been malnutrition of the elderly and its association with pressure ulcers. Dr. Kaminski published the first papers that reassociated pressure ulcers with hypoproteinemia and redemonstrated that the seriousness of an ulcer parallels the deficiency in serum albumin levels. In addition, he has written many other papers, book chapters, manuals, and audiovisual materials. He serves on a large number of editorial boards and is a member of numerous professional societies.

Mildred G. Kemp, PhD, RN, CETN, FAAN
Associate Professor, College of Nursing
Rush University
Practitioner/Teacher, Department of Operating Room and Surgical Nursing
Rush-Presbyterian-St. Luke's Medical Center
Chicago, Illinois
Dr. Kemp is a Certified Enterostomal Therapy Nurse. She has been principal investigator or coinvestigator on several projects targeting the prediction or prevention of pressure ulcers. Her work has been published in the *Western Journal of Nursing Research*, the *Journal of Enterostomal Therapy*, and *Research in Nursing and Health*, and she has presented her research findings on numerous occasions. She is a reviewer for the *Journal of ET Nursing*.

Thomas A. Krouskop, PhD
Professor, Department of Physical Medicine and Rehabilitation
Baylor College of Medicine
Director of Rehabilitation Engineering
The Institute for Rehabilitation and Research
Houston, Texas

Dr. Krouskop's research has encompassed the etiology of pressure ulcers, the mechanics of support surfaces, and noninvasive methods to detect soft tissue damage caused by mechanical loading. He is on the editorial board of the *Journal of Tissue Viability* and serves as a reviewer for the *Archives of Physical Medicine and Rehabilitation, Journal of Biomechanics,* and *Journal of Rehabilitation Research and Development.* In recognition of his contributions to pressure ulcer research, Dr. Krouskop was the 1993 recipient of the Kosiak Award, presented by the National Pressure Ulcer Advisory Panel.

Victor L. Lewis, Jr., MD, FACS
Associate Professor of Clinical Surgery
Northwestern University Medical School
Chicago, Illinois

Dr. Lewis is Associate Professor of Clinical Surgery in the division of Plastic Reconstructive and Maxillo-facial Surgery at Northwestern University Medical School. For the past 17 years, he has been the plastic surgery consultant for the Midwest Regional Spinal Cord Injury Care System at Northwestern Memorial Hospital, Chicago, Illinois. During this period, he has examined several hundred patients with soft tissue complications of spine trauma and has a wide operative experience in the area. Dr. Lewis is the author of multiple publications in the area of pressure sore reconstruction and the evaluation of the bone underlying pressure sores.

JoAnn Maklebust, MSN, RN, CS
Clinical Nurse Specialist, Wound Care
Case Manager for General and Reconstructive Surgery
Harper Hospital, Detroit Medical Center
Detroit, Michigan

Ms. Maklebust is coauthor of the 1991 textbook *Pressure Ulcers: Guidelines for Prevention and Nursing Management.* She serves as legislative chairperson of the National Pressure Ulcer Advisory Panel, is on the editorial board of *Advances in Wound Care*, and is a member of the Wound Healing Society. She has conducted research and published many papers on pressure ulcers. Ms. Maklebust is chairperson of the Harper Hospital Multidisciplinary Pressure Ulcer Task Force and is a member of the hospital product evaluation committee. She is certified as a Clinical Nurse Specialist by the American Nurses Association.

David J. Margolis, MD, FACP
Director, Cutaneous Ulcer Center
University of Pennsylvania Medical Center
Assistant Professor, Department of Dermatology
School of Medicine, University of Pennsylvania
Philadelphia, Pennsylvania

Dr. Margolis is certified in Internal Medicine and Dermatology. He currently has a dermatology practice, is Assistant Professor in Dermatology at the University of Pennsylvania School of Medicine, and is a Fellow of The American Academy of Dermatology and of The College of Physicians of Philadelphia. Dr. Margolis is a member of the Wound Healing Society and is on the board of the National Pressure Ulcer Advisory Panel. He has published and presented papers on chronic wounds, including one on definitions and guidelines for assessing wounds, and the evaluation of healing. He has been a peer reviewer for *Archives of Dermatology, Journal of American Academy of Dermatology, Tissue Repair and Regeneration,* and *Journal of Dermatologic Surgery and Oncology.*

Elena M. Marvel, MSN, MA, RN
State Coordinator, Health Advocacy Services Program in New Jersey
American Association of Retired Persons
Short Hills, New Jersey

As the State Coordinator for the American Association of Retired Persons Health Advocacy Services Program in New Jersey, Ms. Marvel has been involved in health promotion for older adults and Hispanic Outreach in New Jersey. Ms. Marvel has spent her professional career in nursing education and primary care of the aged. She has developed and produced instructional materials using a wide variety of media. She has been a faculty member at Seton Hall University, William Paterson College, and County College of Morris, New Jersey. Ms. Marvel is a member of the board of directors of the New Jersey National League for Nursing; the gerontology advisory council of Rutgers University School of Social Work, Continuing Education Program; and the advisory board of the Northeast Region National Coalition of Hispanic Health and Human Services Organizations (COSSMHO) National Hispanic Leadership Initiative on Cancer project. She served on the 1993 Gubernatorial Transition Team in New Jersey.

Steven I. Reger, PhD, CP
Director of Rehabilitation Engineering, Department of Physical Medicine and Rehabilitation, Department of Plastic Surgery, Department of Biomedical Engineering
The Cleveland Clinic Foundation
Cleveland, Ohio

Dr. Reger is actively involved in biomedical engineering and rehabilitation, with academic appointments, numerous publications, and research grants, especially in the area of tissue load management. He is the first-named on a patent for computer-aided prescription of specialized seats for wheelchairs and other body supports.

George T. Rodeheaver, PhD
Professor and Director of Plastic Surgery Research
Health Sciences Center, University of Virginia
Charlottesville, Virginia

Dr. Rodeheaver has been the director of the Wound Healing Research Laboratory since its creation in 1972. The primary focus of his active research program is wound management and optimization of wound healing. He has published two books, 29 chapters in books, and 154 papers on various aspects of managing wounds. He is president of the National Pressure Ulcer Advisory Panel, is a founding member of the Wound Healing Society, and serves on the editorial board of *Wounds*.

Richard (Sal) Salcido, MD, FAAPMR
Interim Chairman, Department of Physical Medicine and Rehabilitation
Associate, Department of BioMedical Engineering
Associate, Sanders-Brown Center on Aging
University of Kentucky
Cardinal Hill Hospital
Lexington, Kentucky

Dr. Salcido serves on a multidisciplinary pressure ulcer task force in a 100-bed rehabilitation hospital and has been active in education in the area of rehabilitation medicine. The major focus of his funded research is to develop an understanding of fundamental basic science issues with respect to the formation of pressure ulcers. Dr. Salcido was the first recipient of the Bio-Sonics Award for Innovations in Pressure Ulcer Research. He has published and presented extensively on the subject of pressure ulcers, including his work on the role of free radicals in the development of pressure ulcers in an animal model and pressure ulcers in the elderly.

George C. Xakellis, MD
Director of Research and Medical Development
John Deere Health Care Corporation
Moline, Illinois
Dr. Xakellis was an Associate Professor in the Department of Family Practice at the University of Iowa College of Medicine during the development of this guideline. He recently assumed a position at the John Deere Health Care Corporation as Director of Research and Medical Development. Dr. Xakellis is a Fellow of the American Academy of Family Physicians and a member of the Society of Teachers of Family Medicine. He has a Certificate of Added Qualifications in Geriatrics. His research areas are pressure ulcers and evaluation of clinical practice guidelines and their impact on care. Dr. Xakellis is a peer reviewer for *JAMA, Archives of Family Medicine*, and *American Family Physician* and is a grant reviewer for the Family Health Foundation.

Gary M. Yarkony, MD, FAAPMR
Vice President for Clinical Development
Schwab Rehabilitation Hospital and Care Network
Associate Professor of Clinical Physical Medicine and Rehabilitation
Northwestern University Medical School
Chicago, Illinois
Dr. Yarkony is active in practice, education, and research in rehabilitation medicine. He is the Vice President for Clinical Development at the Schwab Rehabilitation Hospital and Care Network. Previously he was the director of rehabilitation for the Midwest Regional Spinal Cord Injury Care System and is a Fellow of the American Academy of Physical Medicine and Rehabilitation. He has numerous publications, lecture series, and presentations on the subject of pressure ulcers, especially with regard to hydrocolloid dressings, Marjolin's ulcers, and pressure ulcers in the elderly. He has served as a peer reviewer for *JAMA, Paraplegia,* and the *Archives of Physical Medicine and Rehabilitation* and as a grant reviewer for the National Institute on Disability and Rehabilitation Research.

Consultants

Richard M. Allman, MD
Associate Professor of Medicine
Director of the Center for Aging and the Division of Gerontology and Geriatrics
University of Alabama at Birmingham
Chief of Geriatrics Section
Birmingham Department of Veterans Affairs Medical Center
Birmingham, Alabama
Pressure Ulcer Treatment Consultant

Ronni Chernoff, PhD, RD
Professor, Nutrition and Dietetics
College of Health Related Professions
University of Arkansas for Medical Sciences
Associate Director, Geriatric Research Education and Clinical Center
John J. McClellan Memorial Veterans Hospital
Little Rock, Arkansas
Nutrition Consultant

Sue Crow, MSN, RN
Nurse Epidemiologist
Associate Professor of Medical Administration
Louisiana State University Medical Center
Shreveport, Louisiana
Infection Control Consultant

David C. Hadorn, MD
RAND Corporation
Santa Monica, California
Clinical Algorithm Consultant

JoAnne Horsley, PhD, RN, FAAN
Professor, School of Nursing
Oregon Health Sciences University
Portland, Oregon
Research Utilization Consultant

Henry Miller, PhD
President
Center for Health Policy Studies
Columbia, Maryland
Economics Consultant

Mary Susan O'Brien, PhD
Professor
Omaha Metropolitan Community College
Omaha, Nebraska
Consumer Consultant

George T. Rodeheaver, PhD
Professor and Director of Plastic Surgery Research
Health Sciences Center
University of Virginia
Charlottesville, Virginia
Wound Care Consultant

Steven H. Woolf, MD, MPH
Assistant Clinical Professor
Department of Family Practice
Medical College of Virginia
Senior Advisor
U.S. Preventive Services Task Force
Washington, District of Columbia
Methodology Consultant

Panel Staff

Janet Cuddigan, PhC, RN
University of Nebraska Medical Center
Omaha, Nebraska
Panel Manager and Research Analyst

Joan Ronnenberg, MSN, RN
University of Nebraska Medical Center
Omaha, Nebraska
Research Analyst

Brenda Bergman-Evans, PhD, RNC
University of Nebraska Medical Center
Omaha, Nebraska
Research Analyst

Elizabeth Gavin
University of Nebraska Medical Center
Omaha, Nebraska
Panel Secretary

Editorial Support

Brenda Bergman-Evans, PhD, RNC
College of Nursing
University of Nebraska Medical Center
Omaha, Nebraska
Scientific Writer for Consumer Version

Morris A. Magnan, MSN, RN
Clinical Nurse Specialist/Case Manager
Critical Care/Cardiology
Harper Hospital, Detroit Medical Center
Doctoral Student
Wayne State University
Detroit, Michigan
Scientific Writer for Consumer Version

JoAnne Maklebust, MSN, RN, CS
Clinical Nurse Specialist for Wound Care
Case Manager for General and Reconstructive Surgery
Harper Hospital, Detroit Medical Center
Detroit, Michigan
Scientific Writer for Consumer Version

Mary Sieggreen, MSN, RN
Clinical Nurse Specialist/Case Manager
Vascular Surgery
Harper Hospital, Detroit Medical Center
Detroit, Michigan
Scientific Writer for Consumer Version

Joyce Black, MSN, RN
College of Nursing
University of Nebraska Medical Center
Omaha, Nebraska
Scientific Writer for Debridement and Operative Repair

Diane Q. Forti, BA
Dedham, Massachusetts
Scientific Editor

Library Services

Kristine Scannell, MLS
Supervisory Librarian
National Library of Medicine
Bethesda, Maryland

Ione Auston, MLS
Supervisory Librarian
National Library of Medicine
Bethesda, Maryland

Catherine Selden, OHSRI
National Library of Medicine
Bethesda, Maryland

Nancy N. Woelfl, PhD
Professor and Director
McGoogan Library of Medicine
University of Nebraska Medical Center
Omaha, Nebraska

Contract Support

Sharon Sokoloff, PhD
Mikalix and Company
Waltham, Massachusetts

Demie Lyons, RN, NP
Mikalix and Company
Waltham, Massachusetts

Marcia R. Feinleib
Technical Resources International, Inc.
Rockville, Maryland

AHCPR Staff

Douglas B. Kamerow, MD, MPH
Director, Office of the Forum for Quality and Effectiveness in Health Care

Carole Hudgings, PhD, FAAN
Senior Health Policy Analyst

Margaret Coopey, MGA, RN
Project Officer

William N. LeVee
Managing Editor

Karen Carp
Product Manager

Peer Reviewers[1]

Roberta S. Abruzzese, EdD, FAAN
Editor, *Advances in Wound Care*
S-N Publications
Garden City, New York

Elaine Jensen Amella, MA, RNCS
Assistant Clinical Instructor
Clinical Nurse Specialist in Gerontology
Division of Nursing
New York University
New York, New York

Edna Atwater, RN
Past President, Dermatology Nurses Association
Duke University Medical Center
Durham, North Carolina

Elizabeth A. Ayello, MS, RN, CS, CETN
Assistant Editor, *Advances in Wound Care*
Clinical Instructor of Nursing
Division of Nursing
New York University
New York, New York

Jettie J. Bailey, BSN, RN, CETN
Enterostomal Therapy Nurse
Visiting Nurse Association of Greater Kansas City
Kansas City, Missouri

Michele Ballou-Hansen
Vice President
H.F. Systems, Inc.
Los Angeles, California

Stephen C. Biondi
Vice President of Clinical Services
United Health, Inc.
Milwaukee, Wisconsin

Steven B. Black, MD, FACS
Medical Director
Clarkson Centre for Wound Healing
Omaha, Nebraska

Barbara Braden, PhD, RN, FAAN
Professor
School of Nursing
Creighton University
Omaha, Nebraska

Rosalind Breslow, PhD, RD
Senior Nutritionist
Westat
Rockville, Maryland

C. L. Brown, RPh, MBA, FASCP
Vice President
Genesis Medical Services
Pittsburgh, Pennsylvania

Susan Brown-Goebeler, MS, RN
Clinical Nurse Specialist, Gerontology
Morristown Memorial Hospital
Morristown, New Jersey

Ruth Bryant, MS, RN, CETN
Consultant
Oklahoma City, Oklahoma

---

[1] These individuals provided peer review. Their participation does not necessarily imply endorsement of the guideline.

Wallace H. J. Chang, MD
Professor of Plastic Surgery
University of Washington
Reviewer for the American Society of Plastic and Reconstructive Surgeons, Inc.
Seattle, Washington

Betty R. Clark, BSN, MEd, RN, CRRN
Manager, Nursing Education
The Institute for Rehabilitation and Research
Houston, Texas

Beverly Clark, BSN, RN, CETN
ET Nurse
Sinai Hospital
Detroit, Michigan

M. Ellen Connerton, MSN, RN
Patient Care Supervisor
Home Health Services of Lee
Cincinnati, Ohio

Roberta Coopersmith, BS, RN
EFS Healthcare Group, Inc.
Chestnut Ridge, New York

Penny S. Crawford, BSN, RN, CETN
ET Nurse
Wound Ostomy and Continence Nurses Society
Norfolk, Virginia

Hilda Curet, MSN, RNC
Nursing Instructor
Veterans Affairs Medical Center
Fort Howard, Maryland

Linda Elena Dallam, MS, RN, GNP
Nursing Services Associate
Montefiore Medical Center
Bronx, New York

Sharon L. Darkovich, BSN, BA, RN
Quality Assurance Coordinator
Metrohealth Saint Luke's Medical Center
Cleveland, Ohio

LeBaron W. Dennis, MD
Reviewer for the American Society of Plastic and Reconstructive Surgeons, Inc.
San Antonio, Texas

Suellen DeWitt, MS, RN
Clinical Nurse Specialist
Wound Healing Center
Medical College of Virginia
Richmond, Virginia

Dorothy Doughty, MS, RN, CETN
Program Director
ET Nursing Education Program
Emory University
Atlanta, Georgia

William H. Eaglstein, MD
Chairman and Harvey Blank Professor
Department of Dermatology and Cutaneous Surgery
University of Miami School of Medicine
Miami, Florida

Paula Erwin-Toth, MSN, RN, CETN
Manager, Enterostomal Therapy Nursing
Director, ET Nursing Education
Cleveland Clinic Foundation
Cleveland, Ohio

Susan Finn, PhD, RD
President
The American Dietetic Association
Chicago, Illinois

Steve B. Fisher, PA-C
Research Physician Assistant
Department of Rehabilitation Medicine
University of Kentucky
Lexington, Kentucky

Evonne Fowler, MN, RN, CETN
Kaiser Bellflower Hospital
Bellflower, California

Kenna S. Given, MD
Professor and Chief
Section of Plastic Surgery
Medical College of Georgia
Reviewer for the American Society of Plastic and Reconstructive Surgeons, Inc.
Augusta, Georgia

Margaret Goldberg, MSN, RN, CETN
Enterostomal Therapist
Crozer-Chester Medical Center
Upland, Pennsylvania

Sharon E. Goldsby, BSN, MS, CRRN
Senior Community Health Nurse
Rehabilitation Specialist
Visiting Nurse Association of Southeast Michigan, East Region
Warren, Michigan

Davina J. Gosnell, PhD, RN, FAAN
Dean and Professor
School of Nursing
Kent State University
Kent, Ohio

Michele Gottschlich, PhD, RD, CNSD
Director, Nutrition Services
Shriners Burns Institute
Cincinnati, Ohio

Martin Grabois, MD
Professor and Chairman of Physical Medicine and Rehabilitation
Baylor College of Medicine
Houston, Texas

Robert H. Graebe
President
ROHO, Inc.
Belleville, Illinois

Peggi Guenter, MSN, RN, CNSN
Nurse Member
American Society for Parenteral and Enteral Nutrition
Silver Spring, Maryland

Charles Gulas, PT
Physical Therapist
Associated Rehabilitation Services/ Rehabilitation Choice
St. Charles, Missouri

Beverly G. Hampton, MSN, RN, OCN, CETN
Director, ET Nurse Education Program
Division of Nursing
University of Texas
M.D. Anderson Cancer Center
Houston, Texas

Michelle Hardaway, MD
Clinical Assistant Professor
Department of Plastic and Reconstructive Surgery
Wayne State University
Attending Surgeon
Harper Hospital/Detroit Medical Center
Detroit, Michigan

Ann H. Harris, MSN, RN, CS
Wound Management Consultant
Independent Practice
Spring Lake, Michigan

Allen W. Heinemann, PhD
Associate Professor
Department of Physical Medicine and Rehabilitation
Northwestern University Medical School
Director, Rehabilitation Services Evaluation Unit
Rehabilitation Institute of Chicago
Chicago, Illinois

Patricia A. Hercules, MS, RN
Manager
Department of Nursing Education
The Methodist Hospital
Houston, Texas

Barbara M. Hergenrother, MAT, RN, CETN
Enterostomal Therapy Nurse
RN Clinician
Visiting Nurse Association of Baltimore, Inc.
Baltimore, Maryland

Sue Hrim, RN
Vice President
Ultra-Med, Inc.
Avoca, Pennsylvania

Katherine F. Jeter, EdD, ET
Executive Director
Help for Incontinent People
Staff Affiliate Enterostomal Therapy
Spartanburg Regional Medical Center
Spartanburg, South Carolina

Kay Jewell, MD
Medical Director
Health Care Financing Administration
Baltimore, Maryland

Jeffrey L. Kaufman, MD
Division of Vascular Surgery
Baystate Medical Center
Springfield, Massachusetts

Joyce Keithley, DNSc, FAAN
Professor
College of Nursing
Rush University
Chicago, Illinois

John C. King, MD
Assistant Professor
Department of Rehabilitation Medicine
The University of Texas Health Science Center at San Antonio
San Antonio, Texas

Luther C. Kloth, MS, PT
Associate Professor
Physical Therapy Department
Marquette University
Milwaukee, Wisconsin

Diane Krasner, MS, RN, CETN
ET Nurse Consultant
Graduate Student
School of Nursing
University of Maryland
Baltimore, Maryland

Thomas A. Krouskop, PE, PhD
Professor
Baylor College of Medicine
Houston, Texas

Betsy Antenucci Kuhn, MSN, RN
Clinical Nurse Specialist
Cleveland Clinic Foundation
Cleveland, Ohio

Margaret M. Landry, RN, CETN
Clinical Resource Specialist
H. F. Systems, Inc.
Los Angeles, California

Diane K. Langemo, PhD, RN
Professor
College of Nursing
University of North Dakota
Grand Forks, North Dakota

Gerald Lazarus, MD
Dean
School of Medicine
University of California, Davis
Medical Sciences Institute of California
Davis, California

Cheri H. Leonard, PA-C
Physician Assistant
Department of Neurology
Brockton Veterans Affairs Medical Center
Brockton, Massachusetts

Monte J. Levinson, MD, CMD
Medical Director
The Presbyterian Homes
Evanston, Illinois

Carol Lingner, RN
Wound Management Coordinator
Deaton Specialty Hospital
Baltimore, Maryland

Clare M. Logan, PA-C
Physician Assistant
Department of Geriatric Medicine
University of Cincinnati Family Medicine
Cincinnati, Ohio

Dennis J. Lynch, MD
Chairman, Department of Surgery
Professor of Surgery
Texas A&M University Health Science Center
Scott & White Clinic
Reviewer for American Society for Plastic and Reconstructive Surgeons, Inc.
Temple, Texas

Morris A. Magnan, MSN, RN
Clinical Nurse Specialist and Case Manager
Harper Hospital, Detroit Medical Center
Doctoral Student
Wayne State University
Detroit, Michigan

Janice Malett, MPH, RN, CETN
Wound/Ostomy Clinical Nurse Specialist
Nyack Hospital
Nyack, New York

Karl A. Matuszewski, RPh, MS
Director
Technology Assessment Program
University Hospital Consortium
Oakbrook, Illinois

Frederick M. Maynard, MD
Medical Director
Metro Health Center for Rehabilitation
Case Western Reserve University
Cleveland, Ohio

Linda McDonald, MSPH, RN, CIC
President
Association for Practitioners in Infection Control
Seattle Veterans Affairs Medical Center
Seattle, Washington

Donald McHale, RN
National Sales Manager
Medical Education Director
Derma Sciences
Old Forge, Pennsylvania

Donna McMullen, RN, CETN
Medical-Surgical Clinician
Shady Grove Adventist Hospital
Rockville, Maryland

Carol Mikols, MSN, RNCS, CETN
Clinical Nurse Specialist
Mid-Michigan Visiting Nurses Association
Midland, Michigan

Paulette Nardi, MT (ASCP), MBA, MICP
Director of Special Projects
National Patient Care Systems
East Rutherford, New Jersey

Kathleen M. Neill, DNSc, RN
Assistant Professor
School of Nursing
Georgetown University
Washington, District of Columbia

Eric Noss
President
Vantage Therapeutics, Inc.
Exton, Pennsylvania

Adrian M. Oleck, MD
DMERC Medical Director
Region B
Indianapolis, Indiana

Sudhir Pahwa, MS, MBA
Vice President Home Care, NASL
Support Systems International
Charleston, South Carolina

Carole H. Patterson, MN, RN
Associate Director for Product Development
Department of Standards
Joint Commission on Accreditation of Healthcare Organizations (JCAHO)
Oakbrook Terrace, Illinois

Carol Peltier, BS, RN
Executive Director
Kansas City Hospice
Kansas City, Missouri

Tania J. Phillips, MD
Associate Professor of Dermatology
Department of Dermatology
School of Medicine
Boston University
Boston, Massachusetts

Bernadette Pohlmann, MS, RNC, CRRN, CPHQ
Clinical Nurse Educator
Quality Improvement Coordinator
Department of Veterans Affairs
Edward Hines, Jr., Veterans Affairs Hospital
Hines, Illinois

Michael M. Priebe, MD
Assistant Professor
Department of Physical Medicine and Rehabilitation
Baylor College of Medicine
Veterans Affairs Medical Center
Houston, Texas

Martin Robson, MD
Chairman, Division of Plastic Surgery
University of Texas Medical Branch at Galveston
Galveston, Texas

Ignatius Daniel Roger, MD
Catholic Medical Center
Forest Hills, New York

Bonnie Sue Rolstad, BA, RN, CETN
Enterostomal Therapy Nurse Specialist
Director
ET Nurse Consultants, PA
St. Paul, Minnesota

Salah Rubayi, MD, FACS, FICS
Clinical Assistant Professor of Surgery
University of Southern California
Chief
Pressure Ulcer Management Service
Rancho Los Amigos Medical Center
Downey, California

Barbara Sadler, BSN, RN, CETN
Enterostomal Therapy Nurse
University of Illinois Hospital
Chicago, Illinois

C. Andrew Salzberg, MD
Assistant Professor of Plastic and Reconstructive Surgery
New York Medical College
WCMC Burn Center
Valhalla, New York

Mary Sandrik, BSN, RN, CETN
Enterostomal Therapy Nurse
Mount Sinai Hospital Medical Center of Chicago
Chicago, Illinois

Martha J. Satwicz, MSN, RN
Quality Specialist
Catherine McAuley Health System
Nursing Development Services
St. Joseph Mercy Hospital
Ann Arbor, Michigan

Freddi Segal-Gidan, PA
Physician Assistant
School of Medicine
University of Southern California
Los Angeles, California
Rancho Los Amigos Medical Center
Downey, California

Sam Shekar, MD, MPH
Executive Medical Director
Office of Coverage and Eligibility Policy
Bureau of Policy Development
Health Care Financing Administration
Baltimore, Maryland

Mary Sieggreen, MSN, RN
Clinical Nurse Specialist/Case Manager
Patient Services, Vascular Surgery
Harper Hospital, Detroit Medical Center
Detroit, Michigan

Carol Smith, MPA, RNC
Service Line Manager, Geriatrics
Geriatric Center
University of Nebraska Hospital
Omaha, Nebraska

Philip W. Smith, MD
Hospital Epidemiologist
Clarkson Hospital
Omaha, Nebraska

Wyonna Stiffler, BSN, RN, CETN
Private Practitioner
Kettering, Ohio

Nancy A. Stotts, MN, EdD
Associate Professor
Department of Physiologic Nursing
University of California
San Francisco, California

Robert Tallon, MD, MBA
DMERC Medical Director
Region C
DMERC Operations
Columbia, South Carolina

Susan S. Thomason, MN, RN, CS
Clinical Nurse Specialist
James A. Haley Veterans Hospital
Tampa, Florida

Elaine Trefler, MEd, OTR, FAOTA
Assistant Professor
Department of Orthopedic Surgery
University of Tennessee, Memphis
Memphis, Tennessee

Pamela G. Unger
Physical Therapist
Unger Physical Therapy
Kutztown, Pennsylvania

Lia van Rijswijk, RN, ET
Consultant
Newtown, Pennsylvania

Carey Vinson, MD, MPM
Medical Utilization Director
Family Health Center Director
Forbes Health System
Monroeville, Pennsylvania

Joseph J. Walsh
Executive Vice President
Derma Sciences, Inc.
Old Forge, Pennsylvania

Deborah Warner, MS, ARNP, CS, CETN
Enterostomal Therapy Clinical Nurse Specialist
St. Joseph's Hospital
Tampa, Florida

Doreen A. White, BSN, RN, CETN
Certified Enterostomal Therapy Nurse
Independent Practice
Springfield, Ohio

Audrey Witko, BSN, RN
Clinical Manager
Huntleigh Healthcare
Manalapan, New Jersey

Michael Wood, MD, FACS
Clinical Associate Professor
Department of Surgery
Wayne State University
General Surgeon
Harper Hospital/Detroit Medical Center
Detroit, Michigan

Kristy Wright, MBA, RN, CETN, FAAN
President
Wound, Ostomy, and Continence Nurses Society
Costa Mesa, California

Robert Zone, MD
DMERC Medical Director
Region D
Nashville, Tennessee

Pilot Review Sites[2]

A. Holly Patterson Geriatric Center
Uniondale, New York
Holly Lidowski, MSN, RN, CNAA

Baptist Medical Centers
Birmingham, Alabama
Martha M. Patrick, MSN, RN

Beatrice Community Hospital
Beatrice, Nebraska
Maggie Spilker, MSN, RN

The Cleveland Clinic Foundation
Cleveland, Ohio
Karen A. Gelliarth, BSN, RN, CETN
Betsy Antenucci Kuhn, MSN, RN

Harper Hospital
Detroit, Michigan
Pilot Implementation
Morris A. Magnan, MSN, RN
JoAnn Maklebust, MSN, RN, CS
Mary Sieggreen, MSN, RN

Living Centers of America
Houston, Texas
Barbara Baylis, MSN, RN

Magee Rehabilitation Hospital
Philadelphia, Pennsylvania
Beth W. Jacobs, RN, CRRN

Methodist Hospital
Houston, Texas
Patricia A. Hercules, MS, RN
Marcia Hill, MS, RN

Methodist Hospital of Indiana, Inc.
Indianapolis, Indiana
Shelley Lancaster, MSN, RN, CS

Mid-Michigan Visiting Nurse Association
Midland, Michigan
Carol Mikols, MSN, RNCS, CETN

Nassau County Medical Center
East Meadow, New York
James T. Evans, MD, FACS

[2] These agencies provided pilot review. Designated agencies also conducted a pilot implementation or case analysis of the guideline. The site coordinators are listed for each pilot review agency. Agency participation does not necessarily imply endorsement of the guideline.

New England Deaconess Hospital
Boston, Massachusetts
Philip Basile, MD
Vivian Seide, MS, RN, CS

Saint John's Queens Hospital
Elmhurst, New York
Patricia M. Dooley, RNC

Silver Cross Hospital
Joliet, Illinois
Sharon Baranoski, MSN, RN, CETN

South Mississippi Home Health, Inc.
Hattiesburg, Mississippi
Sharon Lucy, MS, RN

Strong Memorial Hospital
University of Rochester Medical Center
Rochester, New York
Review and Case Study Analysis
Diane Breton, MS, RN, CRRN

Thomas Jefferson University Hospital
Philadelphia, Pennsylvania
Nancy Tomaselli, MSN, RN, CETN

United Health Inc.
Somerset, Kentucky
Stephen C. Biondi, MS
Norma Jean Griffin, ADN, RN
Cindy Headley, RN
Rebecca Knapp
Robin Patterson, BSN, RNC, NHA
Rita R. Roedel, MS, RN
Nancy J. Watts, BSN, MS

University of Cincinnati Hospital
Cincinnati, Ohio
Arlene C. Miller, MSN, RN, CNS

University Geriatric Rehabilitation Unit
University of Nebraska Hospital Geriatric Center
Omaha, Nebraska
Carol Smith, MPA, RN

University Hospital
University of Nebraska Medical Center
Omaha, Nebraska
Judith J. Warren, PhD, RN

Veterans Affairs Medical Center
Seattle, Washington
Richard Buhrer, MN, RN, CRRN

Visiting Nurse Home Health Services
Warren, Michigan
Sharon E. Goldsby, MS, BSN, RN

Visiting Nurse Association of Omaha
Omaha, Nebraska
Karen S. Martin, MSN, RN, FAAN

Walter Reed Army Medical Center
Washington, District of Columbia
Jean M. Reeder, PhD, RN, FAAN

Attachments

Attachment A. Sample Pressure Ulcer Assessment Guide

Patient Name: ______________________________ Date: ____________ Time: ____________

Ulcer 1:
Site ________________
Stage[a] _______
Size (cm)
Length _______
Width _______
Depth _______

	No	Yes
Sinus Tract	☐	☐
Tunneling	☐	☐
Undermining	☐	☐
Necrotic Tissue	☐	☐
Slough	☐	☐
Eschar	☐	☐
Exudate	☐	☐
Serous	☐	☐
Serosanguineous	☐	☐
Purulent	☐	☐
Granulation	☐	☐
Epithelialization	☐	☐
Pain	☐	☐

Surrounding Skin:

	No	Yes
Erythema	☐	☐
Maceration	☐	☐
Induration	☐	☐

Ulcer 2:
Site ________________
Stage[a] _______
Size (cm)
Length ______
Width _______
Depth _______

	No	Yes
Sinus Tract	☐	☐
Tunneling	☐	☐
Undermining	☐	☐
Necrotic Tissue	☐	☐
Slough	☐	☐
Eschar	☐	☐
Exudate	☐	☐
Serous	☐	☐
Serosanguineous	☐	☐
Purulent	☐	☐
Granulation	☐	☐
Epithelialization	☐	☐
Pain	☐	☐

	No	Yes
Erythema	☐	☐
Maceration	☐	☐
Induration	☐	☐

Description of Ulcer(s):

____

____

Indicate Ulcer Sites:

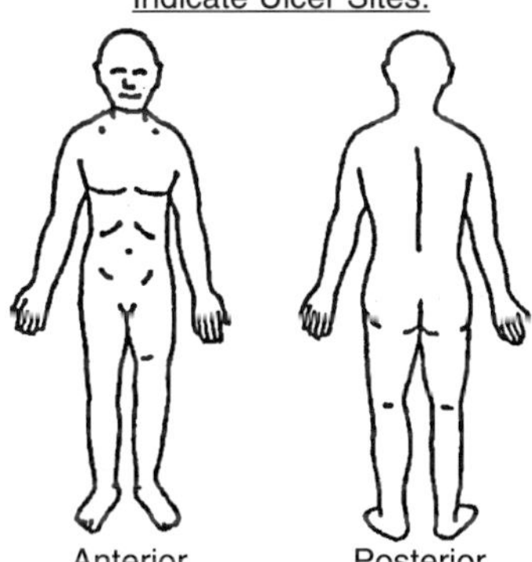

(Attach a color photo of the pressure ulcer[s] [Optional])

[a]Classification of pressure ulcers:

Stage I: Nonblanchable erythema of intact skin, the heralding lesion of skin ulceration. In individuals with darker skin, discoloration of the skin, warmth, edema, induration, or hardness may also be indicators.

Stage II: Partial thickness skin loss involving epidermis, dermis or both.

Stage III: Full thickness skin loss involving damage to or necrosis of subcutaneous tissue that may extend down to, but not through, underlying fascia. The ulcer presents clinically as a deep crater with or without undermining adjacent tissue.

Stage IV: Full thickness skin loss with extensive destruction, tissue necrosis, or damage to muscle, bone, or supporting structures (e.g., tendon or joint capsule).

Attachment B. Sample Nutritional Assessment Guide for Patients With Pressure Ulcers

Patient Name:__________________________Date: _________________Time: _________

To be filled out for all patients at risk on initial evaluation and every 12 weeks thereafter, as indicated. Trends will document the efficacy of nutritional support therapy.

Protein Compartments

Somatic:

Current Weight (kg) _____
Previous Weight (kg) _____ (_____date)
Percent Change in Weight _____

Height (cm) _____
Height/Weight _____
Current Body Mass Index (BMI) _____ [wt/(ht)^2]
Previous BMI _____ (_____date)
Percent Change in BMI _____

Visceral:

Serum Albumin _____
(Normal $\geq$ 3.5 mg/dL)
Total Lymphocyte Count (TLC) _____ (optional)
(White Blood Cell count x percent Lymphocytes/100)

Guide to TLC:

- Immune competence — $\geq$ 1,800 mm^3
- Immunity partly impaired — < 1,800 but $\geq$ 900 mm^3
- Anergy — < 900 mm^3

State of Hydration

24-Hour Intake_______ mL 24-Hour Output _______ mL

Note: Thirst, tongue dryness in non-mouth-breathers and tenting of cervical skin may indicate dehydration. Jugular vein distension may indicate overhydration.

Estimated Nutritional Requirement

Estimated Nonprotein Calories (NPC) _____ /kg Estimated Protein ______ (g/kg)

Actual NPC _____ /kg Actual Protein ______ (g/kg)

Recommendations/Plan

1.
2.
3.
4.

Attachment C. Oral and Cutaneous Signs of Vitamin or Mineral Deficiencies

Clinical Signs (by Site)	Deficiency(ies)
Oral Cavity	
Cheilosis and angular stomatitis	Vitamin B_2
Glossitis (i.e., pink or magenta discoloration with loss of villi)	Multiple B vitamins
Eyes	
Scleral changes	Vitamin A
Bitot's spots	Vitamin A
Face	
Seborrhea-like dryness and redness of nasolabial fold and eyebrows	Zinc
Upper Extremities	
Purplish blotches on lightly traumatized areas (due to capillary fragility and subepithelial hemorrhages)	Vitamin C
Extreme transparency of skin of hands ("cellophane skin")	Vitamin C
Abdomen/Buttocks	
Waxy, perifollicular hyperkeratosis	Vitamin A
Lower Extremities	
Superficial flaking of epidermis, large flakes of dandruff	Essential fatty acids
Cracks in skin between islands of hyperkeratosis:	
■ Pigmented	Nicotinamide (niacinamide)
■ Nonpigmented	Vitamin A

Note: These manifestations may be seen in disease processes other than vitamin deficiencies. If the cause is in fact a deficiency, clinical improvement should be evident 4 weeks after supplementation is begun.

Attachment D. Practical Management of Loose Bowel Movements Related to Tube Feeding

Possible Cause(s)	Treatment
Antibiotic use	Lactobacilli per feeding tube (2 packets tid x 3 doses)
Lactose intolerance	Use lactose-free liquid diet
Choleretic diarrhea	Questran®, 1 g q6–8h and/or Titralac tabs, 2 q6–8h
Mild enterotoxogenic pathogens	Pepto-Bismol®, 30 mL q6–8h
Severe enterotoxogenic pathogens with WBCs in stool on Gram stain	Selected antibiotic per stool culture and sensitivity testing
Insufficient fiber	Fiber supplement, 3 g q6–8h
Idiopathic	Lomotil®, Imodium®, paregoric (Warning: This may cause reactive constipation!)

Note: Any or all treatments may be indicated.
tid = three times daily
q = every
WBC = White Blood Cells

Index

Q

R

S

T

Notes